STO

10·17·79

A Change of Air

By the same author

HERBS THAT HEAL

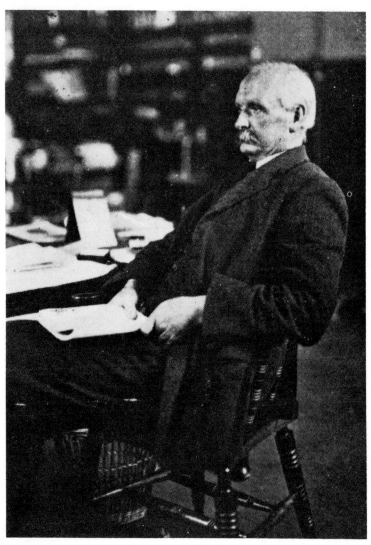

Sir Leonard Hill, F.R.S.

A CHANGE OF AIR

CLIMATE AND HEALTH

William A. R. Thomson, M.D.

CHARLES SCRIBNER'S SONS
NEW YORK

First published 1979 by
A & C Black (Publishers) Limited
35 Bedford Row, London WC1R 4JH

First American edition published by
Charles Scribner's Sons 1979

1 3 5 7 9 11 13 15 17 19   I/C   20 18 16 14 12 10 8 6 4 2

Printed in Great Britain
Library of Congress Catalog Card Number 79-63477
SBN 0-684-16259-8

Contents

Acknowledgements

The author and publisher would like to thank the following for permission to reproduce their illustrations in this book:

Frontispiece Reproduced from 'The Life of Sir Leonard Erskine Hill F.R.S. (1866–1952), Professor Sir Austin Bradford Hill and Mr Brian Hill in the Proceedings of the Royal Society of Medicine, Volume 61, pp. 307–16, March 1968.

Page 23 From Synoptic Climatology, Dr A. H. Perry, in The Climate of the British Isles, Ed. T. J. Chandler and S. Gregory, Longman.

Page 36 Climate, Man and History, Robert Claiborne, Angus & Robertson.

Page 37 A Dictionary of Geography, W. G. Moore, A & C Black Limited.

Page 40 Man, Environment and Disease in Britain, G. Melvyn Howe, David and Charles and Penguin (Pelican).

Page 42 From Radiation and Sunshine, R. H. Collingbourne, in The Climate of the British Isles, Ed. T. J. Chandler and S. Gregory, Longman.

Page 45 Mary Evans Picture Library.

Page 51 A Sketch-Book, Dorothy E. G. Woollard, A & C Black Limited.

Page 57 Swiss National Tourist Office.

Page 61 The Science of Ventilation and Open Air Treatment (Pt II), Leonard Hill, H.M.S.O., 1920.

Page 67 Popperfoto.

Page 73 Popperfoto.

Page 89 Medical Research Council Annual Report 1976–77. Photograph reproduced with the permission of the Controller of Her Majesty's Stationery Office.

Page 109 Courtesy of the Musée de l'Assistance Publique, and Ciba Review Ltd.

Pages 114 & 117 From 'Life and Death of the Solar Topi', E. T. Renbourn, in The Journal of Tropical Medicine No. 65, 1962, Staples and Staples Limited.

Page 119 Journal of the Royal Army Medical Corps No. 102, 1956.

Page 203 Climate, Man and History, Robert Claiborne, Angus and Robertson.

List of illustrations

Dedicated
to
The Memory
of
Sir Leonard Hill, F.R.S.
The Apostle of Fresh Air

Preface

Health is the most potent cause of national prosperity and health depends primarily on weather. Such was the opinion expressed by Ellsworthy Huntington in *World Power and Evolution* some sixty years ago. Yet forty years later one of his fellow-countrymen was bemoaning the fact that 'physicians are taught to use every treatment from penicillin to the scalpel, except the omnipresent climate and weather – or protection from it.' Today this moan is more justified than ever. Surgeons become ever more audacious, whilst physicians use more and more esoteric drugs. But less and less attention is devoted to the effect of climate on the prevention and alleviation of disease. It all sounds very rational but it ignores the fundamentals of life. It is as if one built a superb new ship, with wonderful engines and all the navigational aids that science could produce, but ignored the climatic hazards of hurricanes, icebergs and the like.

As Robert Claiborne has put it so cogently in his fascinating *Climate, Man and History*: 'For all our ingenuity and intelligence, for all the resources of energy we dispose of, we are still small and feeble animals in an enormous universe which, if not actively hostile to life is light years away from being hospitable to it. Our planet, insignificant as it is in the cosmic scheme of things, is yet what one of the astronauts so perceptively called it: an oasis. It is the only oasis we know of, or are likely to know of, within the universal desert. It is our survival capsule in the illimitable bleakness of space.'

All the more reason therefore why we should make full use of what the oasis offers us in the way of climate. Over the millenia it is our surroundings, including the atmosphere in all its climatic variations, that have made us what we are. Unless therefore we adjust ourselves to live in harmony with climate we shall suffer, if not perish. Again and again, all down the ages we see mankind struggling with climate, but all to no avail. We are part and parcel of a universe that incorporates all things living, and, unless we realise this and live in unison with our environment (to use the currently popular catchword), we shall never enjoy life and health to the full.

This oneness of man with Nature was much better understood, even if only partially or subconsciously, in the early days of the human race. Indeed, it might also be claimed that climatology was the basis of the practice of medicine. It was as man became more 'civilised', to use a much abused and misunderstood term, that he gradually became more and more independent of his natural surroundings. At least he thought he was becoming more independent, but experience has shown, and is showing, that such independence is one of the great delusions of life.

As René Dubos has so admirably put it in *Mirage of Health*: 'By changing the physical world to fit his requirements – or wishes – he has almost done away with the need for biological adaptation on his past. He has thus established a biological precedent and is tempting fate, for biological fitness achieved through evolutionary adaptation has been so far the most dependable touchstone of permanent success in the living world.'

Thus so far as climate is concerned, man has sinned against Nature in two ways. He has not only refused to respect it, he has also tried to develop independent of it. The futility of his efforts was succinctly summed up by a Cambridge scientist: 'Man's ability to survive in almost every inhospitable place depends more on his capacity to create a hospitable micro-climate than on the capacity of his physiological processes of thermoregulation.'

Such is the background to this book, in which I have attempted to review the effect of climate on health. As already indicated, it is a long, long story – but a fascinating one. Even coming to historically recorded times, a millenium ago the *Lex Frisonium*, or law of the Friesians, imposed a tax for an inflicted wound if it resulted in a weather-sensitive scar. An early appreciation of the adverse effect of climate on the healing process – and, incidentally, a problem that is still with us but has never been solved. I have ranged widely, but not comprehensively. To have attempted the latter would have involved technicalities and a volume of well-nigh unmanageable size – certainly for the lay (non-medical) reader for whom it is intended. The hazards of hot and cold climes, high altitudes and sunshine have been discussed, as well as the association of climate with heart and lung disease, rheumatism, migraine, mental health, and cancer. The practical side has not been overlooked, and the climatic pro's and con's of bracing and relaxing climates, mountain and sea have been included, as well as the problems of clothing, retirement and travel.

Fortunately, it looks as if the orthodox outlook on medical climatology is beginning to alter along the lines I have advocated. In his Milroy Lecture delivered before the Royal College of Physicians of London in 1976, Professor John Pemberton made the salient point: 'If it is accepted that most diseases are the result of a disturbance of the "equilibrium between man and surrounding nature" it follows that research that includes the environmental component is more likely to be successful in uncovering the etiology of a disease and in devising methods of control than research directed to man alone or the environment alone.' That is a balanced point of view with which I would fully agree, and, if Professor Pemberton can persuade his academic, scientific and medical colleagues to follow his advice, then the outlook for suffering humanity will be correspondingly brighter.

But perhaps I might be allowed to end on a more elegiac note by a quotation from a Swiss source. 'In order to survive *Vitis vinifera* [the grapevine] requires certain climatic conditions. These also seem to be important for man's civilization, because all great early cultures with the exception of the Incas developed in similar climatic regions as required for this plant.' A pleasing version of the old adage, *in vino veritas*, with which might well be left the last word.

I

Historical background

'What is it moulds the life of man?
The weather.'

So wrote Charles Kingsley, perpetuating a belief that goes back to the earliest days of man, and echoing the view expressed rather more poetically by Virgil in his *Georgics*:

'Thus when the changeful temper of the skies
The rare condenses, the dense rarefies,
New motions on the altered air impress'd,
New images and passions fill the breasts;
Then the glad birds in tender concert join,
Then croaks the exulting rook, and sport the lusty kine.'

In the more precise language of a modern United States bioclimatologist – to use one of those horrendous synthetic terms with which scientists are cluttering up our vocabulary: 'Early medicine recognised the oneness of man with his environment and the environmental vicissitudes were seen as the cause of pain and sickness.' 'All life on this planet', one of his contemporaries writes, 'is the result of an evolutionary process extending over many millions of years. In the course of this process the anatomical and physiological characteristics of the living tissue have been shaped and moulded by the environmental factors existing on the planetary surface. Today we exist in equilibrium with very narrow ranges of temperature, pressure, radiation intensity and atmospheric gas composition.'

What we have forgotten today is that the very atoms of which we are made come from the Big Bang – to use the modern astronomer's slang term for the Biblical Creation – which created the universe some 18 000 million years ago. In other words we are part of Nature, made of the same material as all life on earth and dependent upon the weather or climate – call it what you will – for our existence.

This is a concept consistently – and, by then current standards, scientifically promulgated by the Hippocratic School of medicine around 400 B.C. One of the sections in what is now known as *The Medical Works of Hippocrates* is entitled *Airs, Waters, Places*, and carries the sub-title 'an essay on the influence of climate, water supply and situation on health.' According to this, in the translation of Chadwick and Mann (1950):

'Whoever would study medicine aright must learn of the following subjects. First he must consider the effect of each of the seasons of the year and the difference between them. Secondly he must study the warm and the cold winds, both those which are common to every country and those peculiar to a particular locality. Lastly, the effect of water on the health must not be forgotten . . .

Thus he would know what changes to expect in the weather and, not only would he enjoy good health himself for the most part, but he will be very successful in the practice of medicine. If it should be thought that this is more of the business of the meteorologist, then learn that astronomy plays a very important part in medicine since the changes of the seasons produce changes in the mechanism of the body.'

In other words, the doctor had to be a meteorologist if he was going to do justice to his patients. Yet, how many medical schools today include bioclimatology in their curriculum? Certainly none in the United Kingdom.

The scientific tools of the Hippocratic School may have been primitive by twentieth-century standards, but their powers of observation were just as good as, if not better than, ours. It is therefore of interest to read the peroration of *Airs, Waters, Places*:

'The chief controlling factors, then, are the variability of the weather, the type of country and the sort of water which is drunk. You will find, as a general rule, that the constitution and the habits of people follow the nature of the land where they live. Where the soil is rich, soft and well-watered and where surface water is drunk, which is warm in summer and cold in winter, and where the seasons are favourable, you will find the people fleshy, their joints obscured, and their tissues watery. Such people are incapable of great effort. In addition, such a people are, for the most part, cowards. They are easy-going and sleepy, clumsy craftsmen and never keen or delicate. But if the land is bare, waterless and rough, swept by the winter gales and burnt by the summer sun, you will find there a people hard and spare, their joints showing, sinewy and hairy. They are by nature keen and fond of work, they are wakeful, headstrong and self-willed and inclined to fierceness rather than tame. They are keener at their crafts, more intelligent and better warriors.'

A view shared by Charles Kingsley, according to whom:

'Tis the hard grey weather
Breeds hard English men.'

And also by Asclepiades (124–56 B.C.), who included Cicero and Mark Antony among his patients. According to him, Ethiopians became old rapidly since their bodies are burned too much by the sun, whereas Britons lived to a ripe old age because they inhabited a cold region. A millenium after the hey-day of the Hippocratic School, the Roman Empire was to bear witness so tragically to the truth of these observations as they fell victims to the onslaught of the Huns and the Goths from the cold and chilly north.

Although the Hippocratic concept of what has been described as 'man-environment' tended to become submerged as the medical profession, true to type, fell for the current fashion, whether this was practical or philosophical, and in due course patients came to be bled, purged or otherwise maltreated on the basis of false theories, the concept never died out completely. After all, how could it as long as there were honest doctors who based their practice on their own observations, and not on some remote philosopher ensconced in his equivalent of the modern scientist's ivory tower?

Thus Celsus (25 B.C.–A.D. 50), whose *De Medicina* is the oldest medical document after the Hippocratic writings, written around A.D. 30, advised long sea voyages and a change of climate for improving health, while Galen (A.D. 130–200), the medical autocrat of the Roman Empire, sent patients to Castellamare, near Vesuvius, as he believed mountain air to be good for tuberculosis. Pliny (A.D. 23–79), the famous naturalist and encyclopaedist, built his villa at Naples so as to secure sunshine at different times of the day, an excellent way of securing air and warmth in a sunny climate. This is presumably one at least of the sources of the old Italian proverb that 'all diseases come in the dark and get cured in the sun.'

The concept, however, was by no means unique to the Hippocratic School. In China, Emperor Huang, or Hwang Ti (*circa* 2650 B.C.), known as the Yellow Emperor, whose *Nei Ching* (Canon of Medicine) has been described as the greatest Chinese medical classic, recorded that heat impaired the heart and that cold was bad for the lungs. He placed much emphasis on the influence of different winds on health, and noted, amongst other things, that in the south the earth was weak, there was much fog and moisture, and rheumatism was the prevailing disease. In the centre of the country, on the other hand, paralysis, chills and fever were rampant because of the flat humid countryside, whereas in the west the inhabitants were fat and energetic.

Indian medicine, too, attached much importance to climate from its earliest days. Thus, Susruta (*circa* 500 B.C.), who has been described as one of the three greatest names in Hindu medicine, distinguished between six seasons of the year, the most dangerous of which was the rainy season from mid-July to mid-September. To avoid this he recommended for king and subjects alike a sojourn in dry places, a practice which, it has been noted, 'gave rise to health resorts where people and members of the healing art flocked.' A prelude to the Delhi-Simla migration of modern times.

As medicine surfaced after the Dark Ages that followed the fall of the Roman Empire, the Arabs provided one of the great reservoirs of medical knowledge, and by no-one was this more brilliantly expounded than by Avicenna (A.D. 980–1037). Known to his contemporaries as 'the Prince of Physicians', and whose *Canon* has been described as 'the most famous medical text ever written', he recommended his tuberculous patients to the mountains of Cyprus – a reputation they still enjoy. Since the introduction of streptomycin and other effective anti-tuberculous drugs, the need for sanatoria has largely disappeared, but in the pre-streptomycin days the isle of Aphrodite enjoyed an enviable reputation for its sanatoria.

From the seventeenth century onwards the role of climate in health played a large part in the teaching and practice of doctors in the United Kingdom. Thus, Richard Mead (1673–1754), 'the princely Mead' according to his contemporaries, and the 'Great Mead' according to a current bibliographer, taught that variations in barometric pressure affected the fluids around man's nervous system. That he was by no means a voice crying in the desert is evinced by the fact that a later contemporary, John Fothergill (1712–80), a Yorkshire quaker, trained at Edinburgh University, whose consulting practice was said to be one of the largest and most lucrative in London, declaring that he 'climbed on the backs of the poor to the pockets of the rich', left among his posthumous works a book entitled *Observations on the Weather and Diseases of London*. Meanwhile, across the Irish Sea, John Rutty (1698–1775) was keeping a continuous record of the weather and diseases of Dublin, which he summarized in *A Chronological History of the Weather, and Seasons, and of the Prevailing Diseases in Dublin*, published in 1770.

To complete this panorama of what might be described as the academic and bibliographical background to climes that heal, it is worthy of note that the credit for the first book on what our Transatlantic friends love to describe as climatotherapy belongs to London, where, in 1841, was published *The Sanative Influence of Climate*. This was followed by a spate of what have become known as medical geographies and atlases of disease. The outstanding one among these was Augustus Hirsch's *Handbuch der historisch-geographiscen Pathologie*, published in two volumes between 1860 and 1864. An English translation of the second edition appeared between 1883 and 1886.

French contributions included Boudin's two-volume *Traité de géographie et de statistique médicale et des maladies endémiques*, published in 1857, and Lombard's *Traité de climatologie médicale*, consisting of four volumes and atlas, published between 1877 and 1880, in which he advocated mountain climes for a multiplicity of diseases. Both these French writings exemplified an increasing tendency to look upon climate as part and parcel of the variegated factors in man's surroundings responsible for his health and the ills to which he was heir. Thus Boudin writes: 'Man is not born, does not live, suffer, die in the same way in different parts of the world. Conception, birth, and life, sickness and death, all change with climate and soil, with the seasons and the months, with race and nationality. These varied manifestations of life and death, of health and sickness, these incessant changes in time and space and with man's origin, constitute the special object of geographical medicine. Its domain embraces meteorology and physical geography [the Hippocratic 'airs, waters, places'], statistical population laws, comparative pathology of different races, the distribution and migration of disease.'

Little did the nineteenth-century authors, at least outside Germany, of these and comparable publications realise the prostitution the concept of medical geography was to undergo in the Hitlerian Reich. It was perhaps inherent in the Teutonic make-up, and just waiting to be aroused and misused as it was when, in 1931, Heinrich Zeiss, a German hygienist, introduced the concept of geomedicine, which all too soon was bastardised to the notorious geopolitics of the Hitler era. This is not the place to describe the sad tale of the Hitlerian degradation of the term, geomedicine, but it was admirably summed up by Arne Barkhuus in his penetrating analysis of 'Geomedicine and Geopolitics' published in January 1945.

'As long as geomedicine is looked upon as the triangulation of medicine in space [as a tool in prognosis, prophylaxis and prevention] it cannot be denied that it holds out many promising possibilities . . . Unfortunately Zeiss and most of the other writers in this field have mixed a laudable attempt at using geographical methods in connexion with problems of public health research, with highly tendentious political writing. One of his papers is entitled "The Need for a German Geomedicine", and further reading confirms one's worst fears. The old "blood and soil" ideas are rejuvenated. *German* destiny and *German* geomedicine are intimately linked. The "biological" defence of the frontiers towards the Soviet Union is the almost holy task of the new "science". If Zeiss still shows some reserve, his students have lost this completely. It is with wonder and a feeling of disappointment that one reads, for instance, a thesis on geomedicine from the Hygienic Institute in Berlin, in which the writer's only interest is to make political propaganda.'

It is refreshing to turn from this degradation of the healing art to the bludgeoning of interest in climes that heal that inspired both doctors and patients alike in Britain during the Victorian and Edwardian eras. Such was the interest aroused that at a meeting of the Royal Medical and Chirurgical Society on 14 May 1889, it was resolved: 'That a scientific committee be appointed for the purpose of investigating questions of importance in reference to the climatology and balneology of Great Britain and Ireland.' And a high-powered committee it was, carrying out its duties with meticulous care, and covering the whole of the United Kingdom. Its report, *The Climate and Baths of Great Britain*, came out in two volumes: the first, 'The Climates of the South of England, and the Chief Medical Springs of Great Britain', in 1895; the second, 'The Climates of London, and of the Central and Northern Portions of England, Together with Those of Wales and Ireland', in 1902. 'The climates of Scotland', the preface to volume II notes, 'have been omitted, as the committee failed to secure the necessary local information'; a concise factual statement, behind which must be an interesting story which, alas, history fails to record.

It is a quite fascinating book, based upon careful observation, obtained at first hand and by what is now known as questionnaires, but more aptly described as 'circular letters which were sent to the medical men practising at the various health resorts and bath-places.' An interesting example of the change of terminology and of the thoroughness with which the work was done are the 'Notes on the Meteorological Data included in the Tables published in the Report' by the 'Senior Computer to the Royal Meteorological Society', the human predecessor of the vast expensive calculating machines that modern medicine, science and industry demand to carry out what are now looked upon as chores, but were then considered fit matter for human attention. Frequent reference will be made to it in subsequent chapters, but four quotations from the chapter on Cornwall may here be given as samples of the style in which it is written.

'A line drawn from any point of the northern coast, nearly at right angles to it, will reach land first in North America, having traversed two thousand miles of ocean.' (How more concisely and impressively could one depict the exposed nature of this popular stretch of coast-line?)

'The leading influences of the place are wind and sea; in some exposed places on the coast, as at Tintagel, the tomb-stones require to be supported by buttresses lest they should be blown down.'

'The movement and force of the sea is shown by the height to which the surf rises when the waves strike the cliffs, often forming columns 200 feet high . . . The sounds of the sea also give evidence of its influence. Even at its smoothest, when the surface is generally unbroken, a deep undertone presents itself . . . When rough the sea makes itself heard several miles inland.' (Obviously not a part of the country for the weak at heart or those of poor constitution. Rather a perfect example of a bracing climate *in excelsis*.)

'St. Ives is a port and fishing town of much antiquity and little modern enlightenment. The narrow streets are evil-smelling, and the vicinity of the harbour equally so. The town can scarcely be recommended, whatever may be said of spots in the vicinity.'

But one more quotation must be allowed for those who are not aware of the one-time reputation as a health resort of what is nicely described as 'the greatest agglomeration of human beings in the world.'

'London was perhaps once a sanatorium for malarial cases from Essex. St. Earconwald, bishop of the East Saxons, was buried early in the seventh century in his cathedral of St. Paul. The litter in which he was carried about when too ill to walk or ride was placed there, and a visit to his tomb has

9

cured many sick East Saxons. It is reasonable to suppose that a stay on the healthy upland of Ludgate Hill, while performing devotions at St. Earconwald's tomb, was a natural cure for the tertian fever of the Essex marshes . . . Pilgrim Street, leading into Ludgate Hill, was the old way from the landing-place near the mouth of the Fleet, to St. Paul's, and to the tomb of St. Earconwald. When I lived at St. Bartholomew's Hospital, I often looked at the name of Pilgrim Street with interest, as the memorial of a time when Ludgate Hill and St. Paul's Churchyard were a health resort, about which anaemic East Saxons might be seen walking, enjoying the dry soil and fresh air, paying their respects to St. Earconwald, and refreshed more and more every day by the breeze from the hills of Hampstead and Highgate.'

But it was not only the doctors who were sold on climes that heal. Patients, too, had fallen for them in an increasingly big way since Dr Wittie first sang the praises of Scarborough around the time of the Restoration of the Stewarts to the throne: a convenient starting point for what might be described as the modern era of medical climatology. While originally it was the benefits of the home climate that were extolled, the merits of continental climes soon came to the fore. One of the first to propagate their healing powers was Dr Tobias Smollett, who was one of the earliest protagonists of the Riviera as a health resort. Indeed, so far as the Riviera is concerned, he might be described as the discoverer of its healing propensities. Granted that Henry Fielding had made the same trip nine years earlier for the sake of his health, it was Smollett with his superb account of his trip, *Travels Through France and Italy*, published in 1766, who put the Riviera on the British medical map.

It was in 1763, he records, 'I packed up my little family in a hired coach, and attended by my trusty servant, who had lived with me a dozen of years, and now refused to leave me, took the road to Dover, in my way to the south of France, where I hoped the mildness of the climate would prove favourable to the weak state of my lungs.' Whether he had tuberculosis is problematical. He himself refers to his 'bad state of health, troubled with an asthmatic cough, spitting, slow fever, and restlessness.' He kept a detailed 'weather register' which he summed as: 'There is less wind and rain in Nice than in any other part of the world that I know; and such is the serenity of the air, that you see nothing above your head for several months together, but a charming blue expanse, without cloud or speck . . . This air being dry, pure, heavy, and elastic, must be agreeable to the constitution of those who labour under disorders arising from weak nerves, obstructed perspiration, relaxed fibres, a viscidity of lymph, and a languid circulation.'

His experience, however, was not so fortunate in his second winter in Nice when, between November and March, they had fifty-six days of rain which, he adds, 'I take to be a greater quantity than generally falls during the six worst months of the year in the county of Middlesex.' His summing up was:

> 'Were I obliged to pass my life in it, I would endeavour to find a country retreat among the mountains, at some distance from the sea, where I might enjoy a cool air unmolested by those flies, gnats, and other vermin, which render the lower parts almost uninhabitable. To this place I would retire in the month of June, and there continue till the beginning of October, when I would return to my habitation in Nice, where the winter is remarkably mild and agreeable.'

Smollett's high opinion of the Riviera climate was confirmed by an equally distinguished fellow-Scot, Lord Brougham, one of the founders of the 'Godless' University College of London, who first visited the Riviera in 1834, and fell so in love with it that he spent most of his latter days in Cannes when Parliament was not sitting. What helped to bring home to his fellow-countrymen – on both sides of the Tweed – the sunniness of the Riviera, was his report that in Cannes on only three days out of 111 was he unable to perform experiments he was carrying out on light, whereas at

Brougham Hall in Westmorland, there were only three days out of 111 on which he *could* perform them.

One of the many invalids attracted to the Riviera was Dr J. H. Bennet, who had developed pulmonary tuberculosis. He arrived in Mentone in 1859, recovered, instead of dying as he had expected, and set up in practice. Fifteen years later he expressed the view that 'there is a greater probability of pulmonary tuberculosis being arrested, of life being prolonged, and even of a cure being eventually affected if the patient can winter in the south than if he remains all winter in the north of Europe.' He seems to have practised what he preached and to have become a living example of his dicta, for his programme of life became practising in Mentone in the winter, April and May on holiday exploring the Mediterranean coast, and the summer running his practice in England. One of his many patients was R. L. Stevenson.

By then the Riviera in winter had more or less become a 'Little England', as so delightfully depicted in Patrick Howarth's picturesque *When the Riviera was Ours*. The aristocracy, followed by the professional classes, flocked to it – healthy, hypochondriacs and invalids alike all seeking the sun. Its hey-day persisted until the outbreak of war in 1914. Gradually thereafter its character changed and by 1930 the clientele had largely altered, as well as the clear differentiation between the winter and summer season. By 1945 the old reputation of the Cote d'Azur had changed completely. No longer was it the rendezvous of the nouveau riche and the 'smart set', or the jet set as they are now known. The plebs gradually took over, seeking summer sunshine, the social season became reversed, and the French, with their traditional sacrifice of culture and natural beauty on the hearthstone of financial cupidity, converted one of the loveliest stretches of coastline in Europe into an architectural Hades on earth.

As communication by rail and sea became more comfortable, speedier and more reliable, doctors became more ambitious in their climatic prescriptions for those for whom they considered warm sunny climes were indicated, and those who could afford it were recommended to North Africa, Egypt, Madeira, the Canaries and South Africa. To winter abroad became fashionable, whether well or unwell, and it is an intriguing problem as to who followed whom. Did the well start wintering abroad because of the reputation of such places as Algiers, Luxor and Madeira had achieved as health resorts, or did the socially and financially elite (not necessarily synonymous) set the fashion? Be that as it may, doctors were convinced of the benefits of sunshine and warmth for a host of illnesses, including rheumatism. Tradition, not always a lying jade, has it that when he first developed the rheumatoid arthritis that was finally to confine him more or less to a wheelchair for life, Jesse Boot, the founder of the well-known multiple chemist, was advised by his doctor to winter abroad. This he refused to do as he could not leave his rapidly expanding business for this length of time. Finally, as the disease progressed, he compromised by offering to go to Jersey, perhaps not the sunniest of places, but certainly sunnier than Nottingham: a compromise his doctor accepted as better than nothing. Little did he realise that Jesse Boot's offer to go there, where incidentally he met his wife who was to play such a large part in developing the 'fancy' side of his business, was because he had just opened a branch there, which he wished to inspect personally.

Sunshine and warmth, however, were not the only criteria for health resorts. Mountains, with their clear atmosphere, had for long had an attraction for doctors, and had acquired a reputation as being good for those with lung trouble which, in the Victorian era, as often as not meant tuberculosis, or consumption as it was popularly known from its tendency to consume the patient in its inexorable course, achieving its apotheosis in the dreaded galloping consumption which was the fate of so many of the bright young things of those days. As has already been noted, so long ago as the days of the Roman Empire Galen was recommending the slopes of Vesuvius to his 'chesty' patients. To the Victorian doctor it was the Swiss alps that provided the climatic centre for consumption, and from the mid-1800s onwards a steady stream of tuberculous patients found their way to Swiss sanatoria for longer or shorter periods: an influx which the Swiss, with their characteristic acumen, quickly cashed in on, and from which the Swiss medical profession reaped a rich financial harvest – even bigger than they rope in today from dealing with skiers' fractured limbs.

Not that all the sick and ailing requiring climatic change were sent abroad. Indeed, the majority were referred to health resorts within the British Isles: a tradition which dates back many years. Most of these resorts were at the seaside, and a steady regal procession marks the high standing in which these coastal resorts were held by the medical bigwigs: George III was sent to Weymouth, Queen Caroline to Southend, the Duke of Cumberland to Brighton (admittedly Brighton had other than medical attractions for him), and George V to Bognor (hence the Regis which it now proudly boasts). Inland resorts were not neglected, George Eliot, for example, referring to the 'delicious' air of Harrogate, which Southey extolled even more enthusiastically as 'a fine, dry, elastic air so different from that of Keswick that the difference is perceptible in breathing it', adding that 'the air would, I verily believe, give you new life.'

This belief in climes that heal held sway right up to 1939, particularly where diseases of the heart and lungs and rheumatism were concerned. Thus, in 1935 a London consultant was writing in the *British Medical Journal*:

> 'As a general rule climatic treatment is of vital importance in the successful treatment of patients suffering from arteriosclerotic hypertension. They should be advised to winter, if possible, in a warm climate at a moderate altitude, or, preferably, at sea level; suitable places in England include Bournemouth, Torquay, Sidmouth, Paignton etc. on the south coast; or, if the patient prefers and can afford it, he may winter abroad in Madeira, the Canary Islands, Egypt or Algiers.'

Children, too, were considered to benefit from such climes, especially those of the seaside, a European tradition dating back to the eighteenth century. Convalescent homes were then *de rigeur*, and all major hospitals had such homes, or had access to them, to which they sent many of their patients for a rest and change before returning to work. Those who could afford to pay for their own convalescence were recommended to recuperate at a health resort of their own choice – or selected by their doctor.

But perhaps the outlook of the 1914–39 era is best summarized in the words of Lord Moynihan, the doyen of British surgeons of the era, written in 1916:

'In the treatment of gunshot wounds where the septic processes are raging, and the temperature varies through several degrees, an immense advantage will accrue from placing the patient out of doors. While in France I developed a great affection for the tented hospitals. There is great movement of air, warmth, and comfort; when a sunny day comes the side of the tent may be lifted and the patient enjoys the advantages of open-air treatment. Wounds which were sullen in healing quickly brightened and became clean when exposed to the air and sun. Even in the winter, and in Leeds and Sheffield, we have some patients out of doors day and night. I saw at the 3rd Northern General Hospital a row of beds in the open occupied by ruddy, happy men with quickly healing wounds. I asked many of the patients how they liked the exposure, and all at once replied that they were quite happy and "wouldn't go inside to sleep if they could help it". I am confident we do not sufficiently take advantage of the immense help which open-air treatment can give to patients suffering from the serious wounds of war. I find that wounds clean more rapidly, patients sleep better, eat better, and feel better when they are kept out of doors night and day.'

Alas, as in the case of spas, 1945 marked the end of an era for medical climatology. Science ruled the medical roost, drugs were the answer to disease, or some other form of man-made therapy such as surgery or radiotherapy. Indeed, every form of therapy, except climatotherapy, was in favour. The concept of Nature being of therapeutic value was scoffed at by the up and coming young doctors trained in an atmosphere of materialistic, mechanistic medicine. Slowly, however, the medical wheel is coming round full circle, and the thoughtful doctors in our midst are beginning to realise that Nature has much to offer, and that not the least of her offerings are the climes that heal that are discussed in the following chapters.

2

How climate affects health

'All life on this planet', it has been said, 'is the result of an evolutionary process extending over many millions of years. In the course of this process the anatomical and physiological characteristics of the living tissue have been shaped and moulded by the environmental factors existing on the planetary surface. Today we exist in equilibrium with very narrow ranges of temperature, pressure, radiation intensity and atmospheric gas composition.' Indeed, this relationship of man to his atmospheric environment is what has been described as an 'inexorable and absolute' bond, and for the very simple reason that man requires the atmosphere for his very existence. This bond is direct and indirect. The simplest direct bond is that of oxygen. Without oxygen there can be no life. As is discussed in chapter 5, man can become adapted or acclimatised to the relatively low oxygen pressures of high altitudes, but there is a limit. Above 23 000 feet (7000 metres), a well-known mountaineer has said, 'the climber is like a sick man walking in a dream', while above 30 000 feet life is impossible. An equally vital direct bond is that of temperature. If what is known as the core temperature of the body, which, of course, is several degrees higher than that recorded in the mouth, drops below 90° F. (32.5° C.), consciousness is lost, as it is when the temperature rises to around 110° F. (43.7° C.).

The indirect bond is through the effect of climate on water supplies, vegetation and other forms of terrestrial life. Without these man would die of starvation or lack of water. Water may not be quite as essential to man in so far as he can survive lack of it, even absolute, for a considerably longer period than he can tolerate lack of oxygen. Although this interdependability of man and Nature in all her manifestations is not necessarily of immediate concern in any consideration of climes that heal, it is an aspect that cannot be overlooked – partly because it illustrates the vital role that climate plays in maintaining health.

Indeed, so complex is this integration of man and Nature, and of his dependence upon his surroundings – even in spite of all the so-called wonders of modern science – that the nature of the soil on which our food is grown cannot be neglected, and this in turn may be affected by rainfall. At the present moment we are hearing more and more about so-called trace elements in our food which may be to our good or our detriment. Currently, incurable diseases, such as multiple sclerosis and cancer, are being attributed, at least in part, to some abnormality of foodstuffs in this respect, while there is quite convincing evidence of the lack of elements such as zinc and fluoride causing disease. It is a complex problem, on which too many unjustified statements have been made, but it is obviously one requiring careful investigation. As has been pointed out, 'factors such as rainfall, ease of drainage, and rate of microbial decomposition of the organometallic compounds, all influence the length of time that these compounds [from which the trace elements are derived] remain in the soil before being incorporated into food products or washed into lower soil depths and possibly out into drainage waters.'

On the influence of climate on vegetation there is no need to elaborate, but a study of the animal world indicates the importance in their development of adaptation to their habitat. Thus, in polar regions animals, such as the arctic fox, with their thick fur, can tolerate temperatures as low as $-40°$ C. without having to increase their own heat production to maintain their normal body temperature. Equally typical of these polar animals is their short breeding season (a fortnight in November in the case of reindeer) and their ability to exist on comparatively small amounts of water – a relatively scarce commodity in such frozen regions where the annual rainfall may be as low as 200 millimetres (around 8 inches) a year. Even more striking is the way the camel, which came originally (some three million years ago) from Dakota, has adjusted to desert condition, being able to survive at a temperature of 104° F. (40° C.) for eighteen days without water.

This long-term adaptability of mammals to their environment is now being speeded up in an attempt to feed the multiplying millions of the developing tropical countries. As has been pointed out, in many such areas where land has been considered of marginal economic importance, over-all productivity is regulated mainly by the climate. One of these factors is that the conception rate of many species of domestic livestock is related to what is known as the temperature-humidity index. Hot-humid conditions are associated with lower fertility and also a high loss of the new-born. The new-born calf is just as susceptible to heat as the new-born human babe. This impairment of fertility, probably due to the effect of hot-humid conditions on the pituitary gland at the base of the brain, which controls the production of ova and therefore fertility, is most marked in breeds of cattle originating in temperate climes and transported to tropical conditions. Here is a classical example of the effect of hot climate on the healthy working of the body – a subject further considered in chapter 7.

Equally impressive adaptability to climatic conditions is shown by birds, some desert species of which, fed only on dry seeds, can live without water, and it has been reported that one of these, the budgerigar, has fuel for a 14-hour flight: 'better', as it has been noted, 'than the Jumbo Jet which can only fly for twelve hours.' The mechanism whereby these species of birds have adjusted to their arid surroundings is quite fascinating, including the ability to pass a very concentrated urine, thus conserving water, and even reabsorbing some of this to reduce loss still further.

Insects are also affected by climatic conditions. They are easily upset by lack of water, though excess of it can also have a prejudicial effect. Wind, too, plays a large part in their activity by controlling, not only temperature and humidity, but also their flight migrations. Thus, orientation in mosquitoes involves a visual component. Their flight is only maintained when a visual pattern moves beneath them from front to rear. They fly into the wind if they can maintain a forward movement in relation to the ground pattern. If, however, the wind reaches a critical speed this is not possible and they therefore must either turn and fly with the wind, or settle on the ground.

Even more impressive is the relationship of insect behaviour to cyclonic and anticyclonic pressures, so well known, for example, to bee-keepers, and further discussed later in this chapter (see page 26): an observation which has been confirmed in the laboratory under experimental conditions, where irritability of colonies of insects has been detected during a hurricane even though the temperature and humidity of the laboratory were controlled. Further evidence of the susceptibility of insects to climatic conditions was provided by the swarms of hoverflies that invaded the south of England from the Continent in August 1977. 'Most of them', according to a writer in *The Times* of 29 August, 'are now drowned either on their inward or homeward passage across the seas.' 'The reason for these lemming-like migrations', he added, 'are obscure, but they are probably due to their population explosion, scarcity of food supplies in their home countries, and something in the *climatic conditions*' (the italics are mine).

Man has been equally adaptable, as has been succinctly summarized in the admirable review, *A Survey of Human Biometeorology*, published by the World Meteorological Association: 'Modern man evolved from a hominid called Australopithecus who lived in the semi-arid steppe climate of East and Southern Africa. In the million years of his existence on the Earth, man has ranged into and inhabited hot and cold regions, sea-level areas, and the rarefied atmospheres of high mountains.'

The corollary to this, as pointed out in a report on a symposium on *The Adaptation of Man and Animals to Extreme Natural Environments*, held in the U.S.S.R. in 1970, is:

'For survival an organism must remain in a state of equilibrium with its environment. Each organism has genetically fixed anatomical and physiological qualities which fit it for a particular habitat, but the environment is continually changing, both cyclically and sporadically, and the organism responds physiologically to each of these changes in the environment. The dominant and predictable changes are, of course, the daily and annual cycles in meteorological parameters of the environment. The more obvious and superficial physiological responses to the daily and seasonal changes in the environment, such as changes in body temperature, body weight, subcutaneous fat, coat thickness, etc., have long been studied. It is considerably more difficult to detect, measure and correlate the subtle changes in organs and systems within the body. These things cannot be studied even with the most sophisticated radiotelemetric instruments in the intact organism in its natural environment . . . Clearly there is much to learn when one moves out of the controlled conditions in the laboratory and tries to look at Nature as it really is.'

Looking at Nature as it really is is not quite such a simple matter as it sounds – certainly where climate is concerned. Indeed, it is almost as complex as man himself. Among the factors which go to its make-up are temperature, altitude, barometric pressure, humidity, rainfall (or precipitation as the experts call it), sunshine, wind, and electrical disturbances. All or any of these may affect our health, but what complicates the issue is that not infrequently the individual response to climate is more to weather types than to individual meteorological factors such as, for example, humidity. Quite often these individual responses are associated with weather fronts: these are the boundary lines between different air masses. As shown in the accompanying diagram, five such air masses influence British weather, usefully classified as follows in *The Climate of the British Isles* (edited by T. J. Chandler and S. Gregory):

1. *Maritime Polar*   Cold or rather cold at all seasons. Unstable with bright intervals and showers, especially on windward coasts and over high ground. Cloud and showers die out inland at night and in winter. Originate in the northern part of the North Atlantic.

2. *Maritime Tropical*   Mild in winter, warm and close in summer. Stable air with dull skies, hill and coastal fog and drizzle in windward areas but often bright and sunny in sheltered eastern areas. Originate in the subtropical North Atlantic.

3. *Continental Tropical*   Very mild in winter, very warm in summer. Rain at all seasons. Typically cloudy in winter and thundery in summer. Originate in North Africa and over the Mediterranean.

4. *Continental Polar and Continental Arctic*   Very cold in winter; warm in summer. Cloud and showers, often of snow, along the east coast in winter and spring. Usually mainly dry with clear skies in western areas. Originate over Western Russia and the Arctic Ocean.

5. *Maritime Arctic*   Cool or cold at all seasons. Unstable and showery but with good visibilities. Clear skies on leeward areas. Originate in the polar seas.

It is the meeting of two such masses that produces a front, this being the boundary between them. Where a warm mass is replaced by a cold one, what is known as a cold front develops, which is often accompanied by electrical disturbances. Where a warm air

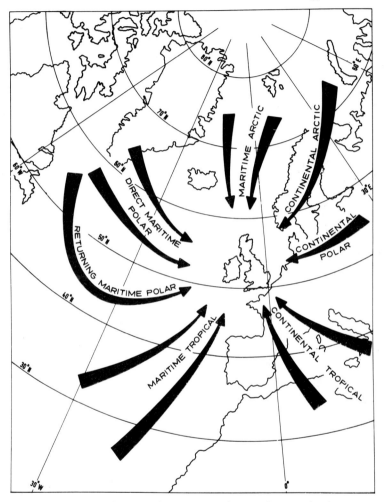

Trajectories of principal air masses affecting the British Isles.

mass, or airstream, pushes against a colder one, a warm front develops.

Correlations of individual responses to weather types are particularly well seen in weather-sensitive patients, those members of the community who are particularly sensitive to climatic changes. They include arthritic subjects and those with scars and amputated limbs. These last were reported on by the distinguished United States neurologist, Weir Mitchell, in 1877 and an extract from this article, which has never been improved upon, gives a perfect picture of what is involved.

'Every storm, as it sweeps across the continent, consists of a vast rain area, at the centre of which is a moving space of greatest barometric depression known as the storm-centre, along which the storm moves like a bead on a thread. The rain usually precedes this by 550 to 600 miles, but before [i.e. beyond] and around the rain lies a belt which may be called the neuralgic margin of the storm, and which precedes the rain by about 150 miles. This fact is very deceptive, because the sufferer may be on the far edge of the storm basin of barometric depression, and seeing nothing of the rain, yet has pain due to the storm.' A state of affairs which he summarizes as: 'A moving area of rain girdled by a neuralgia belt 150 miles wide, within which, as it sweeps along in advance of the storm, prevail in the hurt and maimed limbs of men, and in tender nerves and rheumatic joints, renewed torments called into existence by the stir and perturbation of the elements.' And today, a century later, we know little more about the *modus operandi* of this 'stir and perturbation of the elements.'

Weir Mitchell went on to try and elucidate this problem and once again he is worthy of quotation because of his clarity of thought and because of one of the interesting possibilities he raises:

'A large number of neuralgic attacks seem to be definitely related to the perturbations of the atmosphere which we know as storms. The separate factors of storms, such as lessened pressure, rising temperature, greater humidity, winds, appear as a rule to be incompetent when acting singly to give rise to attacks of pain. Either then it is a combination which works the mischief, or else there is in times of storms, some as yet unknown agency productive of evil. Such an agency may be either electricity or magnetism.'

He then goes on to note that the aurora borealis was 'remarkably brilliant' in 1867 and 1868, and that one of his patients, an army captain with 'neuralgia of a leg stump', who had kept a detailed daily diary for several years of the reaction of his 'neuralgia' to the weather, found his neuralgia to recur during these brilliant displays of the aurora borealis. With his usual caution, Weir Mitchell comments: 'This may be due to magnetic or electrical disturbances, but also it may be owing to the fact that an intense aurora is apt to be followed by a storm.' Even so, this does not rule out the possibility of their being due to what are now known as sferics (see page 26).

This problem of the role of climatic magnetic or electrical disturbances is one that has interested scientists and doctors alike for over two centuries, but opinion is still divided on the subject. There is much anecdotal evidence in support of such disturbances having an effect on man. Thus, it has been claimed that the sensation of freedom felt on mountain tops is due to the high atmospheric electrical potential, whilst the oppression felt in a narrow valley is associated with the virtual lack of electrical tension. As a cynic has commented, however: 'If this "theory" were correct, we would also feel oppressed in a car, in a lovely forest or while swimming.'

It has also been reported, from Germany, that certain individuals who remain for long in the proximity of insufficiently screened radio-wave emitters complain of headache, depression and insomnia. A state of affairs not unlike recent reports from the U.S.A. embassy in Moscow. Another German investigator found marked changes in the threshold of taste during thunderstorms. More convincing is the experiment in which exposure to certain electrical fields induced sensations in weather-sensitive amputees comparable to those they experienced during certain climatic conditions, but not in amputees whose stumps were not weather-sensitive.

These findings are supported by a wealth of experiments on animals and insects. Thus, on days with increased atmospherics (or sferics as they are known for short), which can be simply defined as electromagnetic waves of atmospheric origin, more bees failed to return to their hives than during other weather conditions. Even more impressive were the findings in hamsters. When their nests were exposed to electric alternating fields, within less than forty-eight hours they had moved their nests beyond the range of the field. Mothers with their broods acted even more rapidly. Within twenty-four hours, it is recorded, they 'dragged their young from the field, dismantled the original nest and rebuilt it near the young and transferred the fodder to the new site.' As has been noted, 'these experiments convincingly demonstrate that electric alternating fields, with amplitudes and frequencies comparable to those found in Nature, have a direct biological effect.'

The position today is pretty well that summarised in the following two statements made some ten years ago in a review of the experimental evidence.

'From these experiments we believe it fair to say that these are effects of electric field and electromagnetic radiations at frequencies and amplitudes similar to those found in nature, but none of these warrants the positive conclusion that any biological reaction to the weather may be accounted for by these fields or radiations.'

'By and large current knowledge re the direct effects of electrical alternating fields on man is still sparse and does not admit of final judgments. Nevertheless, we must seriously regard fluctuations of the atmospheric-electricity field, as found in nature, in conjunction with the weather, as likely causal factors in regard to the human organism's reactions, particularly in the light of unequivocal results in certain experiments with animals.'

Those who dislike thunderstorms, however, and wish to take avoiding action may like to know that in the British Isles they are most frequent in May to August, with their highest incidence in the hotter parts of the country. They are relatively infrequent in the west and north-west, especially of Scotland, and the south and east of the Irish Republic.

A more promising development in this field is that of air ions. It was around the turn of the present century that Sir J. J. Thomson, the eminent physicist, demonstrated that air ions are normal constituents of the atmosphere. These may be either large or small, and it is the small air ions that have been attracting increasing attention in recent years. They can be produced artificially, as well as naturally, and the evidence in favour of their action in the whole range of Nature, including man, is now quite impressive. Much of this will be reviewed in subsequent chapters, but meanwhile a brief summary may be given of some of their activities. Thus, in human beings they have been shown to relieve asthma in infants and adults, to have an effect on the brain as demonstrated by electroencephalograms, and to be of benefit in migraine and hay fever. In rats they have a considerable effect on behaviour, while they have an adverse effect on bacteria and viruses, and a beneficial effect on silkworms and growing barley. There is also considerable evidence that the beneficial claims for emanations at certain spas is not due to the radon they contain, but to the ions produced by the action of radon on the atmosphere.

The obverse of all this, which is significant in assessing the effect of climate on the body, and therefore on health, is the variation in the structural and functional features of the natives of different parts of the world. As has been noted, 'though climate is not the only regulatory factor for human body size and proportions, it seems to be the major one'. Thus, we have the big broad build of the Eskimo which allows him to conserve the heat which he

27

generates in his body, compared with the pygmies of the tropical forests, and the linear body build of the desert and savannah inhabitants of the tropics and subtropics. The 'ideal' desert man has been defined as 'linear in build, low in subcutaneous fat, and brunette in colour with high tanning potential', which is an almost exact description of the Solubbies of the Arabian desert, whose heat tolerance is quite exceptional.

Even different forms of heat have different effects on the efficient working of the body. Thus, the Nilotes of the Sudan savannahs are said to be the best adapted inhabitants of the world to hot dry heat, whereas the West African Negro, from whom the United States Negro is descended, has a high tolerance to hot-humid, but not hot-dry, climes. Conversely he has a low resistance to cold, as was shown in the Korean War when Negro G.Is were found to be six times as prone to what are technically known as cold injuries, such as frostbite and the like, as their white compatriots.

This is an illustration of the truth of the *ex cathedra* statement that 'the single most disadvantageous physical property in a healthy individual exposed to a cold environment is early intense peripheral vasoconstriction in the extremities, and a high resistance to release of the vasopasm once it is established'. Which are the characteristics of the Negro, and thus responsible for his susceptibility to cold.

Vasoconstriction, or vasospasm, is the technical word for constriction of the blood-vessels, and occurring in the blood-vessels of the skin it is the body's reaction to exposure to cold. By this means the blood supply to the surface of the body, and particularly those parts of it exposed to the elements, such as the hands, feet and face, is cut down and thereby loss of heat from the body is reduced: a problem more fully discussed in chapter 6. If carried to excess and maintained, it leads in due course to frostbite – or even death.

Those living in arctic conditions, of course, such as Eskimos, have their own built-in methods of adaptation in this, and other respects, to their cold surroundings. This is illustrated, for example, by the fact that they are superior to acclimatized whites in ungloved dexterity under cold conditions. They also have what is known as an increased basal metabolic rate: in other words, an increased production of heat to compensate for the increased loss of heat they sustain in spite of their mode of adaptation to their icy surroundings. It is this increased metabolism which allows them to cope, as one observer has put it, with 'the plentiful fats in their diet, which are enough to sicken most with ketosis.' Even more striking in this respect are the Alacalof Indians of Wellington Island at the tip of South America, who up to a few decades ago wore only otter or seal skins draped over their shoulders. Their basal metabolic rate was so high – up to 200 per cent (the normal in temperate climes is − 15 to + 15 per cent) – that they were able to withstand the chill of repeated diving after seafood in waters of 43° to 46° F. (6° to 8° C.).

This variation in the reaction of man to climate is itself an indication of the important part that climate plays in maintaining health – or inducing disease. The sole purpose of this adjustment, or acclimatisation, is to maintain what Claude Bernard (1813–78), the distinguished French physiologist, described as the 'milieu intérieur', or the internal balance of the cells of which the body is constituted. In the words of his famous aphorism, the fundamental basis of our understanding of the working of the body, 'La fixité du milieu intérieur est la condition de la vie libre, indépendante.' Come war, famine, pestilence, or natural catastrophes, life is ultimately dependent upon the maintenance of this 'milieu intérieur'.

And in essence this in turn is dependent on the water balance of the body. A high content of water is a universal characteristic of living tissues, as exemplified by the fact that nearly 70 per cent of the body, by weight, is water. In other words, the human body is composed of cells, tissues and organs, which contain around 30 litres of water, bathed in some 15 litres of fluid in the form of blood, lymph, and what is known as interstitial fluid: that is, fluid lying between the cells of the body. Whilst the single cell is the functional unit of the body, the human being is not merely a composite of cells, tissues and organs. These, in the words of Pope, are 'but parts of one stupendous whole': an integrated unitary organism. This integration is achieved by means of the nervous system and hormones produced by a series of endocrine glands, such as the thyroid gland, which helps to constitute the Adam's apple in the neck, the pituitary gland which produces a range of hormones, and the adrenal glands which produce cortisone.

As the working of the body is so dependent on the maintenance of the steady state of its internal environment, and this, in turn, is so dependent upon its water content and the distribution of this between the cells of the body and their immediate surroundings, it is clear how climate affects health. If, as already mentioned, the temperature of the body has to be kept steady within certain somewhat narrow limits, then high or low environmental temperatures will have a deleterious effect unless they can be compensated for by the body. As sweating is one of the major means whereby the body adjusts to high temperatures, this means that the humidity of the atmosphere plays an important part in maintaining health. Wind, too, as well as barometric pressure, plays a part, as does the sun, not to mention electrical disturbances or sferics, as has already been outlined.

In addition, there is evidence that atmospheric changes, such as excessive heat, and air ions, affect the production of certain hormones.

The interplay of these factors is still an unsolved jig-saw puzzle, though more and more pieces are falling into place. This, however, is no place to embark on a detailed consideration of these problems that still baffle the scientists – so much so that there is a tendency for them to neglect them in favour of more easily solved problems. The practical aspects of them are discussed in subsequent chapters in so far as they affect health and either induce or ameliorate disease. Much of this information is empirical, based on experience rather than scientifically proven fact – and therefore scoffed at by that school of scientists who wear permanent blinkers. But experience is by no means always a lying jade. Time and again science has in due course confirmed experience. Inevitably it is a rich field for folklore, some of it clearly apocryphal, but much of it well supported by evidence. Its wealth and variety are fascinatingly demonstrated in that classic, fortunately still in print: Richard Inwards' *Weather Lore*.

Be all that as it may,

> 'From Greenland's icy mountains,
> From India's coral strand,
> Where Africa's sunny fountains
> Roll down their golden sand'

as so many of us sang in our childhood's days, man has adjusted to the dictates of climate, and in the course of this adjustment has learned much about those climes that heal that are becoming of increasing interest to the population of the world today.

3

Bracing and relaxing climes

We all talk about bracing and relaxing climates. The terms slip glibly off our tongues, and when we use them we have well-defined specific areas in mind. In practice this works well, and it is a useful classification. In theory, however, they are somewhat difficult terms to define.

Basic to the concept is the important part played by change and contrast. As Sir Leonard Hill pointed out over half a century ago in his monumental report to the Medical Research Council, *The Science of Ventilation and Open Air Treatment*: 'The living substance reacts to the ceaseless play of environment. Its manifestations of energy arise from the transformation of those other forms of energy – heat, light, sound, etc. – which beat upon the transformer, the living substance . . . Of the inflow of sensations which keep us active and alive, and all the organs working in their appointed functions, those from the great cutaneous field are of the highest importance.' In elaborating his theme he evinced that enthusiasm for the open-air life that induced a somewhat esoteric editor of *The Lancet* to describe him as 'the man who invented fresh air', than which no worthier epitaph could be evolved. Some of his typical comments in this context from his Report are worthy of reproduction here as demonstrating dramatically and graphically – possibly, some would contend, exaggeratedly – what this scientist and apostle of fresh air thought about the value of climate in maintaining health.

> 'The salt and sand of wind-driven sea-air and sea-baths act on the skin and brace up the body. The changing play of light, of cold and warmth, stimulate the activity and health of the mind and body. Monotony of occupation and external conditions for long hours destroy vigour and happiness of, and bring about the atrophy of disuse in, men.'

> 'It is the high cooling rate of bracing days which gives the desire for, and joy in, the taking of muscular exercise.'

> 'The ideal conditions out of doors are seen to promote the feeling of comfort and happiness, a gentle cooling breeze to promote adequate cooling of the skin and stimulate the metabolism of the body, coolness and low-vapour tension of air to promote evaporation of water from, and blood-flow through, the respiratory membrane.'

Against this background it is possible to select at least some of the factors that play a part in deciding whether a particular place or area is bracing or relaxing. These are predominantly wind, temperature, and humidity. Change of weather must also be taken into consideration, as well as altitude.

On this basis a bracing climate may be said to be one characterised by dry fresh breezes, a relatively low humidity, a moderately average temperature with a fairly big range between day and night temperatures, and amplitude of sunshine. Conversely, a relaxing climate is one characterised by lack of, or ample protection from, wind, relatively high average temperatures with no great change between nocturnal and diurnal temperatures, fairly high humidity, and ample sunshine.

A complicating factor in Britain is that as often as not our versatile climate refuses to fit into any set, man-made categorisation, so that in any one place it may be bracing at one time and relaxing at another. By and large this is of little significant medical importance, but those who insist on as clear cut a differentiation as possible can often – though by no means always – find what they want abroad, particularly when a relaxing climate is being sought. Again, individual preferences come into the picture; what is bracing to one person may be relaxing to another, and vice versa.

Both these factors are well illustrated in the Riviera. Traditionally it was for long a winter resort where people went to get away from the stormy 'bracing' British winter and obtain warmth and relaxation. But the moment early summer arrived they returned home to Britain in order to avoid the excessive heat and sunshine. Typical of this attitude is the comment of the daughter, and biographer, of Sir David Brewster, Principal of Edinburgh University, who, with her father, spent the winter of 1856–7 in Cannes, when she described the heat in April such as making it 'almost dangerous to move out' between 8 a.m. and 6 p.m. Today the crowds flock to the Riviera in the summer for its warmth and sunshine. Whether such conditions are enervating or relaxing may be a matter for argument, but certainly they could not be described as bracing. Those who seek winter warmth and relaxation in this area, however, run the hazard of a spell of anything but relaxing weather when the mistral blows: a wind which can, and does, cause havoc to the vegetation as well as produce some of the most unpleasant climatic conditions in Europe.

Altitude, temperature, wind, and the relationship to the sea all play a part in determining whether a climate is relaxing or bracing. In temperate zones of the world, such as Western Europe, up to 2000 feet (600 metres) provides a reasonably relaxing climate always provided it is not too exposed to northern winds. Partly this is because such areas are usually well wooded, and trees provide protection from prevailing winds. In passing, it is of interest to note that in temperate zones forest climates have much to be said in their favour for their relaxing or sedative properties. A forest breaks the wind and so plays an important part in temperature control. The atmospheric electrical field is remarkably stable, and the quiet of the forest is soothing to jaded nerves. These attributes of a forest climate were confirmed by a study in and around Munich in 1972, which showed that 'during the summer season forest air is bioclimatically more comfortable than city air for humans.' Traditionally, pine woods have a particularly high repute in this respect. It is certainly true that pine needles dry the earth so that the ground is pleasingly dry, which helps to reduce the humidity of the air, and the branches filter off the solar rays.

Above 3000 feet (900 metres) the climate becomes more bracing, or tonic as some would describe it, whilst anything over 6500 feet (2000 metres) is not recommended for what our continental contemporaries describe as climatotherapy. Conversely a valley climate is essentially relaxing. 2063116

A maritime climate, as it is technically known, is usually bracing, as discussed in chapter 4, but in certain areas it can be pleasantly relaxing.

Warm climes are always relaxing, which explains why our Victorian forbears so sedulously cultivated the warmer parts of Europe and the cooler parts of Africa as alternatives to the bracing hazards of the British climate.

Winds are literally a mixed blessing. They are predominantly stimulating and bracing. On the other hand they can be pleasantly soothing, which is one reason why one seldom feels stuffy at the seaside in hot weather. This is because land heats more rapidly than water. On a sunny summer day therefore ground temperature will soon be higher than sea temperature. As air heated by the hot ground rises (hot air being lighter than cold air) air flows in from the sea to replace it, this giving rise to those cool sea breezes that are so welcome in hot sultry weather. So welcome are they in tropical countries that they are referred to as 'doctor': a tribute to the respect in which the medical profession is still held in at least certain parts of the world. As one writer has put it, 'a still baking morning becomes a breezy cool afternoon.' During the night the converse occurs: the land cools more rapidly than the sea and a land breeze develops blowing offshore. The process is illustrated in the accompanying diagrams.

In this country we have little to complain about our winds, but on the Continent and elsewhere they go in for several thoroughly unpleasant ones. Perhaps the best known of these is the Föhn which

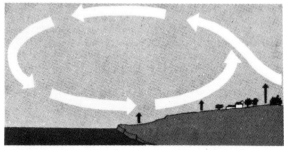

Rapid heating of land generates afternoon sea breeze.

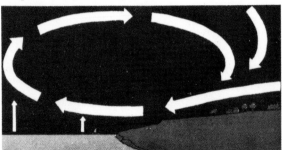

Slow cooling of water produces night-time land breeze.

afflicts mainly the northern Alpine valleys of Switzerland. It is the result of a depression travelling parallel to, and north of, the Alps. This draws in air from the south which disposes of its moisture as rain as it rises over the southern slopes. As it descends the northern slopes it becomes hot and dry. Its hot blast, which will produce a rise in temperature of around 10° to 15° F. (6° to 8° C.), is one of the recognised fire hazards of Switzerland, where a Föhn watch is a statutory obligation on every household. Its effect on health can be quite devastating, including circulatory stress, pain in scars, headache, and giddiness, particularly in the period preceding the Föhn. These human reactions have been attributed to the 'psychological effect of the dramatic natural spectacle, especially when it is connected with fire', but they are nonetheless an unpleasant experience. On the credit side is that in the autumn it helps to speed the harvest, and the grape harvest is largely

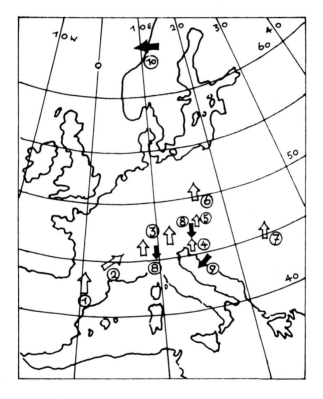

The Föhn winds of Europe: 1 Vent d'Espagne; 2 Vent du Midi; 3 South Föhn of northern Alps; 4 Jauk (Basin of Klagenfurt); 5 Pyrwind; 6 Riesengebirgswind; 7 Roeteturmwind; 8 North Föhn of southern Alps; 9 Bora Adria; 10 Bora of Norway.

dependent on it, while in the spring it speeds the parting snow. Its incidence varies, but in Northern Switzerland it occurs on an average of forty-one days each year, most commonly in the spring and autumn.

Another unpleasant Continental, or, more accurately, Mediterranean, wind is the sirocco, which occurs in winter as the result of a depression entering the Mediterranean through the Straits of Gibraltar and drawing in winds deep from the Sahara. Hot, dry and laden with red dust, it can raise the temperature to over 110° F. (43° C.), producing much bodily and mental discomfort. Offshoot, or after-thought, of it are the mistral in Provence and the bora in the Adriatic. These occur in the rear of the eastern-moving depression as a result of the wind veering to the north-west or north, and causing an icy blast to sweep over Languedoc, Provence and the Riviera in the case of the mistral (literally, 'master-wind', thus indicating the respect, if not fear, of the French for it), and the Adriatic in the case of the bora. A social as well as a health hazard, *The Daily Telegraph* correspondent, covering the wedding of Princess Caroline of Monaco in June 1978, commented: 'The Mistral has struck and it will take all the skill of the Parisian hairdresser Alexandre to keep the coiffures of the bride and her mother in place tomorrow.' The local reputation of the bora was admirably epitomized by Stendhal when he was French consul in Trieste. 'It blows a *bora* twice a week', he wrote in 1831, 'and a high wind on five days. I call it a high wind when I hold on to my hat and a *bora* when I am in danger of breaking my arm.'

Equally well known, though perhaps not quite so forceful, is the famous Cape south-easter which afflicts Cape Town in the summer. This is known as the Cape doctor because it is believed to blow away all the germs. According to Miss Bartha De Blank, however, in her biography of her brother, Archbishop Joost De Blank, 'it is a most tiresome wind and can blow with such strength as to overturn a lorry in the street or sweep people off their feet'. 'It also', she adds, 'brings the cloud down on to Table Mountain – the famous Tablecloth – giving dull and gloomy weather'.

So far as England and Wales are concerned, the distribution of relaxing and bracing climates is shown in the accompanying map. The distribution in Scotland is approximately the same, the western side of the country being relaxing, the east bracing, while, by and large, the Highlands and the Southern Uplands are bracing. In this context, as in so many others, Robert Burns had the right idea when he referred, on the one hand, to the 'cauld blast' from the east that some would say is euphemistically described as bracing, and, on the other hand, wrote:

> 'of a' the airts the wind can blaw,
> I dearly like the west'.

That soothing, mild wind bringing with it the transmitted warmth of the Azores and the gulf stream.

From the map it will be seen that in England and Wales there are four categories of climate inscribed.

1. *Very bracing*   The north-east coast and the High Peak District of Derbyshire.
2. *Bracing*   The rest of the east coast, much of the Sussex coast, and the north coast of Cornwall.
3. *Relaxing*   The south coast of Devon, the west coast of Wales and England, the western half of England sheltered by the Welsh mountains, and the Isle of Wight.
4. *Very Relaxing*   A short stretch on the south-west coast, centred around Falmouth.

This, of course, is only a general guide, and like all general guides it has its exceptions. Thus, much depends on the temperature, and this on average is higher in the south-west coast of England than the north-west coast of Scotland. Equally important is the varying extent to which a place may be sheltered. In South Devon, for example, Budleigh Salterton tends to be rather more bracing than

A Change of Air

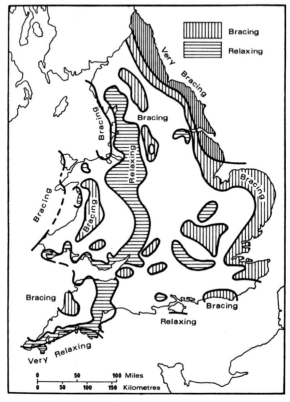

Bracing and relaxing climates in England and Wales (based on Brooks 1954).

the nearby Sidmouth which, as has been said, 'is sheltered from all but the more balmy winds.'

What has also to be borne in mind is the fickleness of the British climate. No matter where one settles, or goes on holiday, some days are more bracing than others, some more relaxing than others. All that can be said is that, on the whole, a place is more relaxing than bracing, or vice versa. What should be insisted on, as

40

Dr Edgar Hawkins pointed out in his book on *Medical Climatology of England and Wales*, published in 1923, is that 'to obtain the full benefit of climate as a therapeutic agent, certain elements should be found in that climate. The air should be pure, free alike from organic impurities, dust, and too much humidity; there should be plenty of bright sunshine without any excess of heat; the temperature should be without extremes; and there should be an absence of violent winds.' To which he adds a forceful affidavit: 'No place can claim to be a satisfactory health resort which cannot show to its credit at least 1500 hours a year of sunshine, of which 500 hours should be in October to March.'

As for which type of climate suits which type of illness we are rather less dogmatic or precise than were the authors of *Climates and Baths of Great Britain*, or Dr Hawkins. One factor that accounts for this is the dramatic change in the outlook for the tuberculous patient produced by the introduction of streptomycin and subsequent anti-tuberculosis drugs. Right up to the middle of this century – that is, little more than a quarter of a century ago – climate played a predominant part in the treatment of tuberculosis in all its manifestations, whether involving the lungs, the bones or the lymph glands. Fresh air in a bracing atmosphere was the basis of therapy. Today these are still the ideal conditions under which an individual should live once his tuberculous infection has been overcome by the appropriate drugs, but there is no reason why he should not live and work anywhere provided his infection has been brought under control, and provided he obeys the elementary rules of healthy living.

What must also be emphasised is that there is no universally favourable climate. The choice must always take into consideration the individual patient, and it is not only his physical state that matters. His whims, as some might call them, must also be borne in mind. There is no point in directing a patient to a place where he is going to be miserable and languishing for comforts, company and conditions not available in the health resort recommended by his doctor. A discontented patient seldom adjusts to life.

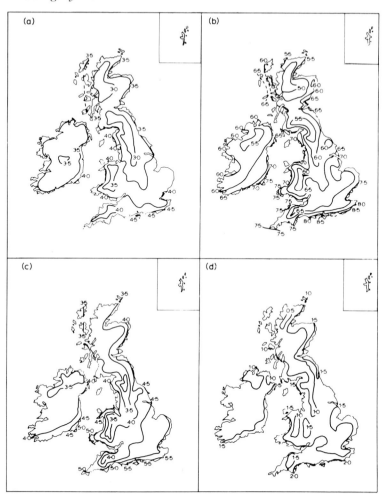

Average daily bright sunshine in hours, 1941–70. (a) March; (b) June; (c) September; (d) December.

In general, relaxing climates are suitable for the elderly, the 'delicate' of all ages, those with heart trouble, subjects of chronic lung trouble such as chronic bronchitis, rheumatic subjects provided the atmosphere is not too humid and the soil provides adequate drainage, the 'highly strung' or neurotic, the tense individual who requires to unwind, and those unfortunates suffering from insomnia.

Bracing climes are indicated for the convalescent who requires 'toning up' after an illness or operation, children who are 'under par', the tuberculous subject who has responded to drug therapy but who is not ready to return to work, the individual, whether business executive, professional man, or housewife who spends most of his (or her) time indoors or in a motor car, for whom a bracing holiday will do a world of good, allowing adequate exercise and mental and physical relaxation.

It will be noticed that what some would regard as somewhat old-fashioned terms, such as 'toning up' and 'under par', have been used. No apology is made for this. The so-called scientific doctors may scoff at them as they are indefinable in precise terms. But the doctor who bases his advice on what he has learned in dealing with his fellow-beings knows exactly what they mean in human terms.

Whether the patient should be advised to make his choice at home or overseas is largely a matter of financial considerations, the patient's own wishes, and whether or not the correspondingly longer journey is advisable. The psychological factor also comes into play. As a world-famous titled statistician once put it: 'The moment I step aboard the boat at Dover I feel better.'

For those seeking relaxing climes – either for permanent residence, a temporary holiday, or to winter abroad – the favourite countries or areas that have stood up to the test of time are the Riviera, North Africa, Madeira and the Canary Islands, Egypt, and South Africa. Medically, the bracing clime of choice is the Swiss Alps in winter, partly because the Swiss, with their traditional nose for business, lay themselves out, medically and hostelry-wise, to cater for those seeking physical and mental rehabilitation.

4

Seaside resorts

There are few natives of this island home of ours who can resist the pull of the sea. This is scarcely surprising, for we are dependent upon it for our livelihood. As two world wars showed, unless Britannia (with her allies) rules the waves, starvation faces us. Until the introduction of air combat and atomic warfare we were dependent upon the sea for our independence, and still proudly boast that for over nine hundred years we have been immune from invasion. We are also dependent upon our sea-girt status, and our geographical situation, for one of the most satisfying and healthiest climates in the world, free from all those hazards of Nature to which so many others are subject such as earthquakes, tornadoes and the like.

All these we take for granted, but it was long before we began to realise and appreciate the health value of our coast-line. A slow beginning was made by Dr Wittie of Scarborough around 1660, whose 'cure' included sea bathing and the drinking of sea water. With its emphasis on the benefits of the bracing north-east winds that swept over what was then nothing more than a bleak fishing village, it was a spartan regime that he imposed on his patients.

Some ninety years later Dr Richard Russell, of Malling, near Lewes in Sussex, gained for himself a permanent, if minor, niche in the medical hall of fame with his dissertation on the uses of salt

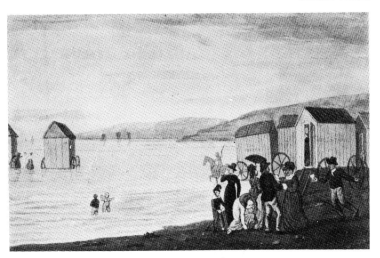

Green's 'Poetical Sketch' of Scarborough: one of a series.

water in diseases of the glands, based on his experience at nearby Brighton, to which he had been attracted by its fine air, and where he continued to practise until his death in 1759. His book was an almost immediate success, and before long, in spite of transport difficulties, 'many invalids', it has been reported, 'came and took his prescription of sea bathing and sunshine' at Brighton. 'Needless to say,' this commentator continues, 'members of the aristocracy and people of fashion set the pace and came in flocks to Brighton. Noteworthy among these were the Duke and Duchess of Marlborough, the Duke of Cumberland ("the butcher of Culloden Moor"), and the Countess of Huntingdon, who sold her jewels to erect a chapel in North Street.' She and John Wesley may have been at daggers drawn over theological matters, but the latter could have had nothing but admiration for Russell's regime.

More importantly from the point of view of medical progress Russell's dissertation was equally influential in medical circles.

Thus, in the summer of 1780 we find Dr Erasmus Darwin, the grandfather of Charles Darwin, sending the sister-in-law of one of his fellow-members of the famous Lunar Society to Scarborough as she was showing symptoms suspiciously like those of her sister who had just died of tuberculosis. The 'Cure' was apparently successful because in December 1780 she married her widowed brother-in-law. Amongst others, whose attention, and approval it attracted, was Dr Lettsom, one of the outstanding London consultants of the time. It was largely through his influence that in 1796 was founded the Royal Sea-Bathing Hospital at Margate, which thus became what has been described as 'a world pioneer for marine hospitals'. Until 1858 it was only open in the summer, but subsequently was kept open the whole year round – and predominantly for children. Writing in 1919, Dr T. D. Luke, in *Spas and Health Resorts of the British Isles*, comments: 'Margate is well known as a resort for tuberculous children, and any morning passing along the Esplanade we see quite a number of pathetic little carriages conveying children kept constantly in the supine position with tuberculous disease of the spine.' A tragic comment on the price our children were having to pay for generations of medical neglect.

Not to be outdone, Scarborough responded to the challenge from the south by building the Royal Northern Sea Bathing Infirmary in 1812. To round off the picture, 1938 saw the opening by the London County Council of the Princess Mary's Convalescent Hospital at Margate, described by *The Lancet* at the time as 'the latest and one of the largest on the coast with accommodation for 223 women and 14 babies in 4-bedded wards and sunny day-rooms.'

Similar moves to make use of the health-giving properties of the seaside followed on the Continent, particularly in Italy, France and Germany. The German marine hospitals were mainly on islands off the North Sea coast, including the island of Föhr, and it is interesting that the first of these was established in 1881 at the request of the Crown Princess (later the Empress Frederick)

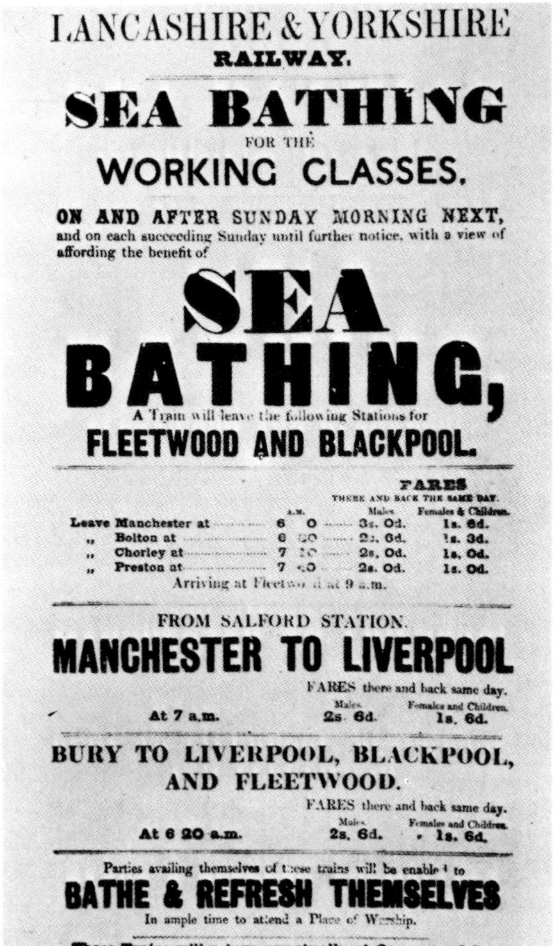

A railway poster of the 1840s advertising sea bathing.

because of its similarity to the Isle of Wight where she had spent so many happy seaside holidays at Osborne. These North Sea hospitals catered mainly for the children of Berlin and Hamburg.

How precisely a marine climate acts is not quite clear. One doctor, with a wide experience on the island of Föhr, like most other writers on the subject, refers to the stimulating effect and the 'stimuli of the seashore' as being 'sun, air, water, winds and waves. These having a stimulating effect on the metabolism of the body in general and on the circulation. In a healthy child at the seaside the capillaries, or small bloodvessels, of the skin react rapidly to climatic stimuli on the skin, whether these be sunshine, wind, cold air, or rolling breaking waves.' 'In pale, weakly and under-nourished children damaged by town life', he continues, 'and sent by health officers or doctors to the seashore, the same reactions occur, but they are slower or weaker.' As a result these unfortunate children feel miserably cold after the shortest sea-bathe, even in August, and even when merely playing on the beach. They cannot tolerate bathing at first, but 'during the cure [using this term in the German sense of a course of treatment] the capillaries gradually recover their normal "gymnastic" function. The circulatory reactions improve week by week, and the same children who felt "terribly cold" and cried at their first bathe could play later on in the open air without clothing, even in stormy weather.' 'At the present time', he adds, 'the children play out of doors for hours, even in winter, and for half-an-hour daily, without clothing. This they do with enjoyment even in the snow.'

A similar picture is painted by that apostle of fresh air, Sir Leonard Hill: 'In the open-air schools of the London County Council, established for weakly children, where good food, rest, and work in the open air are provided, the weight and health of the children increase amazingly. Cases of heart disease, nervous children easily overwrought, those in danger of tuberculosis, those subject to colds and coughs, are alike benefited beyond measure.' He then goes on to describe 'a home for tuberculous children taken from slum tenements, where, unless there is a bitter wind, the children are more or less uncovered. In the winter, after their baths, they run round the sleeping shelter with bare legs and scant attire. In summer weather they go about all day with only knickers on and sleep in canvas shelters. They never show discomfort from cold, or suffer from catarrhs, and come to regard going in as a punishment. Well fed to meet the energy demands, they do extraordinarily well.'

Two other beneficial effects of 'maritime climatotherapy', to give it its ponderous official title, may be briefly mentioned. One is that the cool air and the continual breezes of the seashore deepen breathing and also have a beneficial effect on the lining membrane of the respiratory tract.

All of which has been admirably summed up by a Folkestone doctor. 'The common features of all seaside climates are abundance of light, a pure, warm, moist saline air, an equable temperature, and a dense atmosphere with frequent small barometric differences. All these phenomena stimulate metabolism and are therefore bracing – some more so than others.'

While this 'bracing' factor may be the most important one in maritime medicine, as it is sometimes described, an equal but opposite relaxing action can be obtained, 'slowing down the various vital processes of the body and so economizing the energies of the body', as in resorts on the south coast of Devon, and for some this is what is called for. As has been pointed out, 'there is in England a great variety of local climates. They differ in many ways, such as aspect, shelter, wind, temperature and humidity.' 'No general rule', it is added, 'is therefore possible, for in all climates both stimulant and sedative influences are combined.'

Over forty years ago a leader in the *British Medical Journal* summed up the medical possibilities of our coastline in these words:

'The 6000 miles of seashore of the British Island, with their temperate and invigorating climates, have a great variety of air and shelter, at different seasons, on the North Sea, on the

Atlantic, and on the long range of the south coast. Such a provision of nature is unrivalled in Europe, and suggests large possibilities for the health of a crowded industrial population. It is possible that, especially for the children from towns and cities, something like a national preventive and curative regime might be made available at the seaside, under medical men of special experience and training.'

Some seven years later, in 1938, a committee was set up in London to 'establish centres of research for delicate children on the coast', a move referred to with approbation by *The Lancet*. Alas, it was one of the many victims of Munich and its sequel, and failed to survive the holocaust of 1939–45. The nation was then presented with a National Health Service, so hidebound by convention that the possibility of such a use of the healing properties of our well-nigh unique coast-line was not even hinted at. It is true that holidays with pay have increased the exodus of children and adults of all ranks of society to our seaside resorts, but this is not enough. Unless all the lip-service paid by doctors and officials of the National Health Service to preventive medicine is to rise like the hot air of politicians and disappear into the stratosphere, the 1938 concept of a coordinated service to make full use of the health potentialities of our coasts must be renovated and put into practice.

This should include both research and practice. The full potentialities of a maritime climate have never been investigated on a scientific basis. For instance, what is the difference between 'fresh-air therapy' at the sea and inland? What are the differences between mountain therapy and maritime therapy? The clinical evidence of the benefits of treatment at the seaside has been clear for many years, and these are quite sufficient to justify money being spent on its development rather than on dangerous drugs. At the same time money spent on research in this field, rather than on some of the more exotic fields being ploughed by research workers at the moment, would ensure that we were making full use of this wealth of health-ensuring measures provided by Nature.

Summer holidays by the sea are a step in the right direction, but more is necessary to ensure that all our citizens, particularly children, are obtaining maximum benefit from these. 'I do like to be beside the seaside' sang our Edwardian parents, and how right they were. It is up to their Elizabethan successors to make sure that full use is made of the healing powers of this magnificent coast-line of ours. Britannia may not still rule the waves, but our seafaring instincts should compel us to claim the maximum benefit from this, one of the most valuable uses to which our maritime tradition can be put.

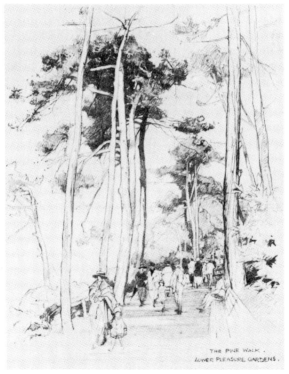

The Pine Walk, Lower Pleasure Gardens, Bournemouth.

5

Mountains and health

'I will lift up mine eyes unto the hills', wrote the psalmist, and there are few of us can resist the call of the mountains. There is a grandeur about them that moves even the most phlegmatic and unemotional in our midst. It is not only the prophets of old who sought inspiration or communion with the Supreme Being on the mountain tops. Their mysteries have tempted the explorers in our midst to physical feats of endurance that have caught the imagination of the public over and over again. Everest is a household name, the conquest of which still inspires international competition.

Medically, too, they have intrigued mankind for many a century, and that they are still a source of perennial interest to the searching mind in medicine is evidenced by the fact that as recently as 1977 two research workers in the Liverpool School of Medicine produced a massive tome entitled *Man at High Altitude*, from which much of the information in this chapter has been acquired. Another equally fascinating source of medical information on the subject, curiously enough, is the result of the Chinese invasion of Tibet. The consequent tension between China and India involved the posting of Indian troops to what must be the highest boundary zone in the world – at 12 000 to 18 000 feet (3650 to 5500 metres). The Indian army medical authorities have taken full advantage of this unique opportunity to study the effect of high altitudes on man, and over the last few years have produced a series of reports which have thrown new light on the subject. Much credit is due to the Indian authorities for seizing the opportunity and to their medical staff for the skill with which they have carried out the task.

Before discussing the use of mountains as health resorts, a review is indicated of some of the main effects of high altitudes on man. The most important of these is the question of oxygen, without which life is impossible. The amount of oxygen in the atmosphere remains constant at 20.93 per cent up to a height of 364 000 feet (110 000 metres), but what matters, so far as man (as well as animals) is concerned, is the *pressure* of oxygen, and this is dependent on the barometric pressure which diminishes with height. What in practice this means is illustrated by one example. At sea-level the barometric pressure is 760 millimetres of mercury, and therefore the pressure, or, more correctly speaking, the partial pressure, of oxygen is 20.93 per cent of this, which is 159 millimetres of mercury. At a height, however, of, say, 11 500 feet (3500 metres), the barometric pressure is down to 493 millimetres of mercury, which means that the partial pressure of oxygen is only 103 : that is, 65 per cent of the sea-level value.

To compensate for this, and ensure an adequate supply of oxygen to the tissues of the body, Nature performs one of her most wonderful miracles. First, there is an increase of around a quarter in the rate of breathing. In addition, there is an increase in the number of red blood cells (technically, erythrocytes) by about a third and in the amount of haemoglobin in the body. The significance of this is that it is haemoglobin, the red pigment in the red blood cells, which is responsible for transporting oxygen from the lungs to all the tissues of the body. Thus by increasing the amount of haemoglobin circulating round the body Nature compensates for the diminished availability of oxygen resulting from its lowered pressure. So sensitive is the body to this lack of oxygen in the atmosphere at high altitudes that within two hours of arrival at a high altitude the production of red blood cells has begun to

53

increase. There is, however, a limit to the extent to which the body can compensate in this way. This is reached at around a height of 19 500 feet (6000 metres), after which there is a decrease in the number of red blood cells and the amount of haemoglobin.

Even more fascinating are some of the other methods whereby Nature compensates for this low pressure of oxygen at high altitudes. One is by increasing the number of small blood-vessels, or capillaries in the lungs. By this means the oxygen in the alveoli, the smallest air-containing channels in the lungs, is brought into close contact with the haemoglobin in the blood, thereby increasing the amount of oxygen it can take up. Having got the maximal possible oxygen to the tissues, Nature then takes steps to ensure that the cells of the tissues make full use of what is available. This is done mainly by increasing the amount of myoglobin. This is the iron-containing substance in the tissues which receives the oxygen from the passing haemoglobin and then makes it available to the cells in which it (the myoglobin) is contained. There is also evidence that other constituents of the cells involved in the complicated use of oxygen are increased. Not only are there these functional changes, there are also structural changes. Thus, the structure of the pulmonary artery, the blood-vessel which carries blood to the lungs from the heart, is altered. As the authors of *Man at High Altitude* point out: 'It is salutary to realise that our anatomy may be modified by the barometric pressure of the air we breathe' and, they might have added, an excellent example of how dependent we are on the climate for our health and welfare.

It is, of course, this lack of oxygen at high altitude that made the conquest of Everest impossible until oxygen was used. This was a measure that was fought tooth and nail by the older generation of mountaineers, such as General C. G. Bruce, who considered it unsporting to make use of such scientific devices. Man must be able to conquer Everest by his own unaided efforts and the oxygen-supplying mechanism with which Nature had endowed him. Optimal physical fitness, ensured by guts, training and experience, was the secret of success, and to attempt to add science to this trilogy was the prostitution of sportsmanship. Scientists, notably Sir Leonard Hill, persisted in pointing out how oxygen breathing apparatus was a *sine qua non* of getting to the top of Everest, but the old guard fought a gallant rearguard action, of which Sir Leonard had a delightful tale to tell.

He was invited to speak at a meeting of the Alpine Club, of which General Bruce was president. In the course of his speech he referred to experiments with oxygen carried out in decompression chambers, in which different altitudes can be simulated in the laboratory, and which are used now on a wide scale in experimental work in deep sea diving and high altitude flying. In thanking Sir Leonard for his speech the gallant general made it perfectly clear that he was still not convinced of the necessity for oxygen to climb Everest, adding: 'As for chambers, I know only of one place for them, and that is under the bed.'

On 8 May 1978, Reinhold Messner, of Italy, and Peter Habeler of Austria, reached the top of Everest without, it is claimed, the use of oxygen. Oxygen, however, was used by the rest of their party. Whether or not this is what might be described as a 'freak' climb is being ardently argued by the experts. Certainly the technique of this pair of climbers was exceptional, and it will be interesting to see whether anyone else can repeat their feat. One possible explanation is that it is now believed that the barometric pressure on the summit of Everest at 29 028 feet (8844 metres) is equivalent to only 27 500 feet (8379 metres) on the standard altimeter scale.

While oxygen supplies are Nature's main concern in ensuring survival at high altitudes, she induces other ancillary methods of adaptation. These include an increased production of essential hormones. There is also an increase in what are known as immunoglobulins – one of the factors responsible for overcoming infections of the body.

In this context it is of interest that the concentration of bacteria decreases with increasing height, and that they are rare above 1600 feet (500 metres). This has been attributed to the small air ions having a lethal action on bacteria and fungi. A study carried out on the Jungfraujoch (13 100 feet [4000 metres]) showed that the number of bacteria in the outdoor air was very low despite the fact that a relatively large number of tourists frequent the area.

Another characteristic is that with increasing height the temperature falls approximately 1° C. for every 500 feet (150 metres). One feature of this is that there can be a striking difference between the temperature in the shade and that in direct sunshine. As one writer has graphically put it: 'You may enjoy a hot cup of coffee while lounging in the sun but if by any chance the shadow of your body falls upon the cup, your drink may be frozen.' To which he adds: 'These quick alterations are as conducive to vigorous life as a monotonous climate is depressing.' It is the same observer who equally graphically draws attention to the effect of the wind at high altitudes. Describing the valley of Findelen above Zermatt, he comments: 'On the slope facing north the vegetation is that of the Siberian tundra, on the other, cereals ripen at an altitude of 6900 feet (2100 metres), and the vegetation is that of the arid and barren tracts on the Mediterranean border. While a well-aimed stone can traverse the geographical distance, the climatic distance is from Iceland to the Rock of Gibraltar.'

In spite of the fall in temperature with height there is increased exposure to solar radiation, including ultra-violet radiation, a problem discussed in chapter 8. The effect of this solar radiation is further enhanced by the clear air of many mountains, which more easily permits the passage of solar radiation to the earth. The effect, most noticeably in the case of ultra-violet radiation, is increased by the reflectivity of snow, which is 75 to 90 per cent, compared with 10 to 15 per cent in the case of ground covered by grass or heather. So far as ionizing radiation is concerned, the authors of *Man at High Altitude* comment: 'It is not possible to identify any deleterious effects due to increased cosmic radiation at high altitude, even though at a height of 9800 feet (3000 metres) there is a three-fold increase in the sea-level value of approximately 24 milliamps per annum of ionizing radiation.' 'The hypoxia [low-oxygen] environment of high altitude,' they add, 'is likely to offer some

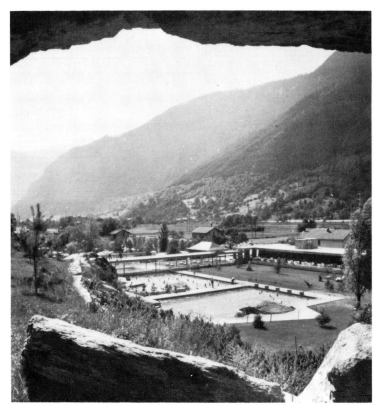

Brigerbad, a mountain health resort in Switzerland.

protection against the level of radiation . . . It seems unlikely that increased environmental radiation at high altitude plays a significant role in the life of the highlanders.' To which they might have added, even less in the case of the visitor.

The only other points that need be mentioned are that there is usually less atmospheric turbulence and water vapour, and often a higher ozone content at high altitudes. And last, but by no means least, in these days of atmospheric pollution, there is a smaller pollutant content of the air.

Inevitably the combined effect of all these climatic and atmospheric changes is quite considerable, varying with the height involved, and the duration of stay. According to the Indian report already referred to, 'prolonged stay at high altitude significantly lowers the incidence of diseases commonly met at sea level.' Among the 130 700 men studied between 1965 and 1972 there was a significantly lower incidence of infection, diabetes, asthma, high blood pressure, coronary heart disease, rheumatoid arthritis, anaemia, stomach disorders, skin disease and psychiatric disease at high altitude than at sea level. The practical implications of some of these findings will be discussed in chapters 12, 13 and 18, dealing, respectively, with heart disease, asthma, arthritis, and mental disease.

Obviously no-one is going to recommend retirement to the high altitudes of the Himalayas or the Andes in order to avoid developing certain diseases but, equally obviously, mountains offer certain definite advantages from the point of view of alleviating such diseases in that vast majority of mankind that lives at or around sea level. The first recorded efforts in mountain therapy as we know it today took place around 1840 in Switzerland, where a treatment centre for scrofulous children was opened at Davos.

This movement spread, steadily gathering momentum, particularly in Switzerland, with the emphasis on the treatment of tuberculosis in all its forms. Here Professor Rollier achieved international fame for his treatment of non-pulmonary tuberculosis, especially of the bones including the spine, which he instituted at Leysin in 1901. I had the privilege of visiting Leysin some fifty years later, by which time it was his justifiably proud boast that he had cured 60 000 cases of tuberculosis. It was an experience I shall never forget. As I wrote at the time:

'Leysin at a height of just over 3000 feet (900 metres) lies in a lovely wooded valley, surrounded by mountains of moderate height which in June [when I visited it] are clear of snow, but across the Rhone there is a magnificent view of the snow-clad Alps. There is a softness about the immediate surroundings that lends an air of intimate peace and quietness to the scene, which is enhanced by the distant background of perpetual snow . . . For the sick patient the combination would appear to be ideal: the softness of the immediate scene encouraging that peace of mind which, even in these days of scientific medicine, is still an essential part of treatment, particularly in chronic conditions such as tuberculosis, whilst the stern yet lovely distant prospect must be a stimulus to the convalescent patient, reminding him of the fuller life he will be able to live when he is finally discharged to his distant home.'

I was particularly impressed by the children's clinic, aptly named La Rose des Alpes, and of this I wrote:

'Here were children from practically every country in Europe, all suffering from various forms and degrees of surgical tuberculosis mainly of the bones and joints: all with beautifully browned and firm bodies, and wearing a minimum of clothing. The majority lay in the ventral posture [i.e., on the stomach] . . . To have been privileged to watch these children carry out their gymnastic exercises to music is an unforgettable experience. With a coordination and rhythm that were a joy to watch, each child performed the prescribed movements so far as his disability would allow. Only one of the children seen on this occasion was able to sit up in bed to perform the full range of movements. Some were able to use all four limbs, some only the lower limbs, some the upper limbs, and one recently admitted child was only able to keep time with lateral movements of her head. But no matter what the disability, every child entered into the drill with a gusto and a genuine pleasure that could not be surpassed. Here, indeed, was a practical demonstration of how the way of the stricken child could be made easy.'

Perhaps I may be forgiven for adding an even more glowing account of a Swiss sanatorium for children, written by a distinguished Swiss doctor. 'The alpine sanatorium offers open-air galleries with light pouring down from the vast open sky, and flooded with air. A beautiful world of snowy peaks and hazy valleys spreads out beyond. Windowless bedrooms with curtains to keep out snow. With a cloth round their loins the children roll about in the dry, sunny, powdery snow. Practically naked, with skin as black as old oak, they snowball one another, skate, toboggan, fly down the slopes on skis.'

Whilst tuberculosis had what might be described as the prior claim on mountain therapy, its scope gradually widened, and today covers an impressive range of conditions. According to one United States authority, the prime indications for mountain therapy are the physically or intellectually overworked, especially if they are strong enough to react to the stimulating effects of climate; convalescents, and those with asthma or chronic bronchitis. In choosing, or recommending, a mountain resort, more care is necessary than in the case of a health resort at or around sea level. In the first instance, invalids seldom do well at heights over 6500 feet (2000 metres). Indeed, in the case of those with heart trouble heights should be avoided; particularly is this the case if there is any evidence of the heart failing.

In this context a warning is necessary in view of the increasing adventurousness of the providers of so-called package tours or holidays – one of the uglier faces of modern democracy. These are now incorporating the more exotic parts of the world, such as high altitudes. This is a subject discussed in more detail in chapter 21, dealing with travel. All that therefore need to be said here is that no-one, however fit, should proceed to high altitudes, say 10 000 feet (3300 metres) or over, except in easy stages. This is because of

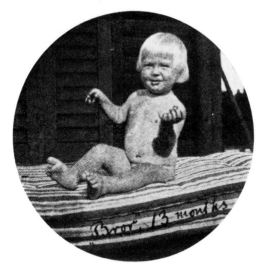

A toddler undergoing open air treatment and daily exercise at a German children's home.

the risk of developing what is known as mountain sickness, an unpleasant, and occasionally fatal, condition which afflicts some people if they climb too quickly, thereby failing to give the body time to adjust to the effects of the lowered barometric pressure and the accompanying lack of oxygen. Even the most experienced mountaineer may be affected by it. Whymper, who achieved fame as the first man to climb the Matterhorn (14 780 feet; 4500 metres) in 1866, suffered from it.

In certain parts of the world, such as the Andes, it is possible to fly from sea level to quite considerable heights in the matter of an hour or so, and such a rapid ascent may well prove awkward, if not serious, for an individual susceptible to mountain sickness, especially if he or she has a defective heart. Unfortunately, it is not possible to judge in advance which individuals will be likely to suffer from mountain sickness, though there is some evidence that those of a nervous temperament are more susceptible to it than the more placid members of society. Indeed, as has been noted, 'individuals of nervous temperament and psychological instability are not likely to do well at great elevation.' And the advice some authorities give is: 'The traveller should not attempt to ascend from sea level to high altitudes rapidly . . . It is much better to break the journey and spend a few days at an intermediate altitude.' To which they add: 'On arrival at a high altitude it is wise not to indulge in too much physical activity on the first few days.'

A final warning note must be struck. In deciding on a mountaineering holiday or convalescence, particular attention must be devoted to the exposure of the selected site. As it has been expressed: 'Distinction must be made between the windy and strong-stimulus windward side and the protected and mild-stimulus lee-side.' The higher one climbs, the more marked is this difference. By and large all mountain holidays are stimulating or bracing – at least anything over 1000 feet (300 metres), but the windward side may be more than has been bargained for. Especially is this so for the highly strung individual, in whom the constant irritation of the wind may induce a condition much worse than that for which relief was being sought. Which, of course, is one reason why a mountain holiday is seldom suitable for those suffering from sleeplessness or insomnia. Fresh air is undoubtedly one of the most valuable of climatic healing forces, but in excess, as on a windy mountain site, it may literally, as well as meta-phorically, prove more than the mortal human frame can tolerate. In other words, we have another variation on the old theme about one man's food being another man's poison. Incidentally, in assessing the curative possibilities of a mountain health resort, a factor that must be borne in mind is that, as has been pointed out, 'a special characteristic of intermediary altitudes is the large number of trees which protect against wind' as well as other climatic factors.

The mountains of the world offer an infinite variety of climatic conditions – almost an embarrassment of riches. They also have their dangers. It therefore behoves the seeker after health to use them with discrimination and with knowledge. Used in this way they can provide some of the most satisfying methods of maintaining, or returning to, health, for which we should all be duly thankful.

6

Hazards of cold climes

'Incredible as it may seem to the well-clad and housed that man should ensure nakedness in winter climate worse than ours, yet Darwin describes this of the natives of Tierra del Fuego [where summer temperatures are around 50° F (10° C.) and winter temperatures around 33° F. (.5° C.) with days as cold as 12° F. (−11° C.)] – the woman with babe at her breast, both naked and the sleet falling and melting on them – the man with at most an otter skin, the size of a handkerchief, worn on the back and laced across the chest and shifted to the side struck by the icy wind. Stunted in growth, with faces hideous with white paint, they sleep on the ground curled up in forms like hares . . . They not only do not decrease in number but they commit infanticide to keep the population down to the food supply.' Such is Sir Leonard Hill's summary of the relevant section of *Voyage of The Beagle*. It was observations such as this that led Darwin to comment: 'Nature by making habit omnipotent and its effects hereditary has fitted the Fuegian to the climate and productions of his miserable country . . . In this wretched climate subject to such extreme cold is it not most wonderful that human beings should be able to exist unclothed and without shelter?'

'In contrast with the naked Fuegians', Sir Leonard pictured 'a curate who visited the laboratory on a mild winter day, and complained that he always felt cold. He wore a thick llama wool vest, a thick woollen shirt, a wool-lined waistcoat, a cardigan jacket with long sleeves, a tweed suit, and a wool-lined covercoat. Why should this guardian of men's souls thus induce the perfect heat-regulating mechanism of his body to atrophy from disuse? Nursery training had instilled into him the fear of cold draughts and wet feet . . . What a range of adaptability of the body habit is there between the curate and the Fuegian.' To which comment he adds: 'So hardy are the Highland soldiers that, wet with snow in wintry weather, they would take off their kilts to dry them on a brazier, and think nothing of standing in the trenches without them.' Sixty years on, when afar and asunder parted are those gallant Highlanders from the gory fields of Flanders, one cannot help wondering: 'Stands Scotland where it did?'

Be all that as it may, these excerpts from the testament of the 'inventor of fresh air' graphically illustrate the incredible ability of the human body to adjust itself to climatic extremes. For all practical purposes, as has previously been noted, for the functional efficiency of the body to be maintained, its core temperature should not fall below 97° F. (36.4° C.). If it falls below 90° F. (32.5° C.) consciousness is lost. This is still compatible with life provided the individual is otherwise fit, the hypothermia, as it is known, is not of long duration, and adequate and efficient treatment is given. Body temperatures of as low as 60° F. (15.5° C.) have been recorded, with recovery.

The body's adaptation to low temperatures consists basically of two procedures: vasoconstriction of the blood-vessels in the skin, and shivering. The vasoconstriction, or narrowing of the blood-vessels, is produced by the same method as their dilatation on exposure to heat: by a reflex action mediated through centres in the brain. This cutting down of the amount of blood flowing through the skin reduces the amount of heat lost from the body to the cold outer air, and thereby helps to maintain the body temperature. It is this vasoconstriction that is responsible for those cold, blue fingers with which we are all acquainted in cold weather

– some of us more than others. Just as the warmth and restoration of normal colour induced by a warmer external temperature as on coming indoors, or rubbing the hands, are due to the blood-vessels dilating up again. Incidentally, it should be noted that, if this re-warming process is carried out too energetically, it may result in quite considerable discomfort.

If this vasoconstriction is marked and sustained for long periods, it may lead to one of the major hazards of cold climes, namely, frostbite. In moderation this is curable but, if extensive or prolonged, it may lead to death of the tissues thus deprived of their vital blood supply, resulting in loss of a finger, toe, foot, hand, or even part of a leg in extreme cases. It is, of course, the extremities of the body that are most liable to frostbite as they are most exposed to the elements. The ears and nose are also vulnerable. A lesser, and much commoner, hazard is chilblains, and here there is a built-in susceptibility. Some unfortunate members of society, more often women than men, develop chilblains every winter, no matter how careful they are about keeping their feet and hands warm, and the younger generation of women found in the early '70s that the craze for miniskirts made them susceptible to chilblains on some embarrassing parts of their anatomy. If only these susceptible members of the community would wear sensible warm clothes and well-fitting footwear, and desist from toasting their toes in front of a lovely warm fire when they come in out of the cold, the incidence of chilblains would fall dramatically.

The other major adaptation of the body to low temperatures is shivering. Unpleasant though this may be, it is an admirable way of helping to maintain body temperature by muscular action, which, after all, is one of the major methods of maintaining normal body temperature. In essence, shivering is comparable to the swinging of the arms, or stamping of the feet that one indulges in on a cold day. Shivering is muscular exercise and it can increase heat production four- or five-fold. In addition there is an increase in the output of two of the important hormones of the body: adrenaline and thyroxine. The latter is particularly important as it

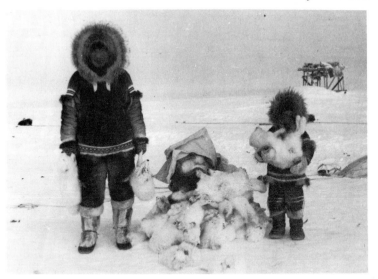

An Eskimo hunter and his young son on Victoria Island.

stimulates the metabolism of the body and thereby its heat production. An interesting side-line of this shunting of energy into heat production is the slower rate of growth of children in cold climes than in temperate climes.

At one time it was contended that a good lining of fat, or adipose tissue, underneath the skin provided an excellent insulation against loss of heat – rather like the double-glazing and other forms of insulation that all of us are being urged to introduce in our houses to reduce the loss of heat and thereby reduce our terrifying bills for whatever form of fuel we may use – whether gas, electricity, coal, or oil. As an example of this we are always being reminded that channel swimmers, no matter what their sex, are well lined in this way. Whilst such a subcutaneous shell of fat undoubtedly contributes to lowering conductivity of heat from the body, this contribution is clearly not as great as was at one time thought. Its heat-insulating power is only about twice that of skin. In this

67

context it is of interest that there is no scientific evidence to justify the old story that Eskimos are well padded with adipose tissue. They are certainly well covered, and their young women would find it difficult to obtain jobs as chorus girls, but as a race they are not particularly fat. It is possibly their facial fat padding that has created this impression.

An adaptive feature that the Eskimos do show is a better blood flow in the hand. Whether this is genetic or acquired after birth is an open question, but it has been shown experimentally that in an ice bath with a temperature of $41°$ F. $(5°$ C.) they maintain a higher surface temperature, as a result of a better blood flow in the hand, than white subjects. Old Crow Reservation Indians have a comparable superior ability to maintain warm hands in cold water. In this context it is worthy of note that the lowest air temperature at which naked men can maintain the core temperature of the body without increasing the metabolic turnover of the body is around $77–81°$ F. $(25–7°$ C.).

Two ancillary factors that often accompany cold and enhance its unpleasantness, if not its dangers, are wind and damp. The baneful influence of wind has always been a point stressed by polar explorers. A century and a half ago, Captain Parry (*Journal of a Voyage for the Discovery of the North West Passage*, 1821), recording a temperature of $-44°$ C., commented: 'Not the slightest inconvenience was suffered from exposure to the open air, by a person well clothed, so long as the weather was perfectly calm; but in walking against a very light air of wind, a smarting sensation was experienced all over the face, accompanied by a pain in the middle of the forehead, which soon became quite severe.'

Nigh on a century later, Griffith Taylor, who was with Captain Scott in the Antarctic, was recording in a diary: 'On the 4th of July, it is a snorting day; wind 50 miles an hour and temperature $-29°$ F. I went out for a few minutes with bare hands, and it took me five minutes in the hut to get them right. Yet it is warmer than yesterday, when bare hands were possible. The wind does it.' On 14 August his entry was: 'Today a beautiful day, with a temperature of − 38° F. (70° of frost) but with no wind, so that one can stay out comfortably.'

'Wind chill,' as this quite disastrous combination of wind and frost is known, has been aptly described as a 'powerful cause of frostbite to nose and ears as well as to penis and digits.'

Is there any truth in the old wife's tale that a damp cloudy day feels much colder than one at the same temperature but with a low humidity? The popular answer is in the affirmative but, as so often happens in the case of such popular beliefs, scientific evidence in its favour is hard to come by. The popular concept is admirably summed up by a Toronto team of investigators who studied the problem in unclothed men, but failed to find confirmation of the traditional belief, though they were careful to point out that 'the effects of humidity on the clothing may be of such importance that the physiological effect seen in unclothed men is of relatively little practical importance.' Their judicial summing up of the popular concept is: 'Field studies, and a great deal of military experience has indicated definitely that the problems of thermal protection of clothed men in the cold, specially at temperatures near freezing point, are much greater when relative humidity is high than when it is low. Damp-cold weather seems to be much "colder" for clothed men than dry-cold, and this is the prevailing opinion from civilian experience also.'

A somewhat more practical test carried out by another Toronto team failed equally to solve the problem. This test consisted of a panel of six commenting on coldness and dampness after walking half a mile (800 metres) at 08.15 hours five days a week for twenty weeks in wintry weather in 'one of the colder parts of Eastern Canada' – and that is saying something. 'The most constant result', it is recorded, was that the panel considered the atmosphere to be dry when the sun was shining irrespective of the relative humidity or total water content. When this factor was allowed for it was apparent that the panellists' predictions of humidity were not very consistent or accurate, but, it is conceded, 'the average of individual comments on dampness did show some slight, and significant, correlation with actual humidity.'

All of which takes us very little further, but one explanation is forthcoming of the term 'damp cold'. At night there is a tendency to condensation, as witnessed, for example, by the formation of dew. Hence the historical concept that 'damp night air' is to be avoided. Further, if the clothes become damp, as by sweating, on a cold day, condensation of this moisture occurs in the outer layer of the clothes, nearest the environment. It was this that led quite naturally though incorrectly, to the assumption that the moisture came from the environment: hence 'damp cold'. To which those schoolchildren who still study Euclid – if such exist today – would say Q.E.D. But the wise doctor will hold his whish.

The most important hazard of cold in temperate climates is hypothermia in the elderly. Hypothermia, which literally means the condition characterised by low body temperature, is occurring with increasing frequency in Britain as our number of elderly citizens increases. Every year brings its toll of death from this entirely avoidable condition, which is fully discussed in chapter 19. It is also a condition that is liable to affect those entering life as premature babies. In them temperature control is far from perfect, indeed scarcely existent in the very premature. This is one reason why they must be nursed in special units where they are not only protected from infection, and have their food and fluid intake carefully controlled, but also have the temperature of their surroundings checked with equal care.

So far as the sick and ailing are concerned, those with heart disease are particularly vulnerable to cold – as they are to heat. Those with chronic bronchitis also find cold climes difficult to adjust to.

Cold in moderation is a wonderful stimulant for the hale and hearty but, like all good things, it must be handled with care. Abused it can, and does, extort a heavy toll of life.

7

Hazards of hot climes

Over two hundred years ago, James Lind, the founder of naval hygiene in Britain, in *An Essay on Diseases Incidental in Europeans in Hot Climates*, published in 1788, emphasised the hazards of heat. As little attention was paid to his views on this subject as was given to those he had put forward fifteen years earlier in *A Treatise of the Scurvy*, in which he urged the issue of lemon juice to the Royal Navy as a preventive against scurvy. But the Senior Service has always tended to display that resistance to new ideas that is said to be one of the attributes of seniority (or senescence, as some would describe it). How many gallant sailors went to a watery grave as a result of Lind's advice in these two reports being ignored is anyone's guess, but practically eighty years after the publication of the *Essay*, three officers and thirty ratings died of heatstroke on the same day aboard the frigate H.M.S. *Liverpool*, proceeding from Muscat to Bushire.

Some seventy years on, as they say in Harrow, in 1911, *The Lancet*, 'inspired' by 'the unusually prolonged heat wave of great intensity that has recently afflicted North America, and which is at present threatening us' (incidentally a heat wave that produced one of the most brilliant of the Edwardian London seasons), evoked a leader entitled 'Sunstroke'. In this it summarised four theories as to its causation. The first was the caloric theory which attributed sunstroke to 'the action of heat *per se.*' This it rejected on the grounds that 'the stokers of the steamships in the Red Sea are scarcely ever affected by the heat of the furnaces.' A statement not in accordance with the facts. The Red Sea was renowned for the strain it put on ships' stokers, and even in living memory it was not unknown for a near-demented stoker to dash on deck and either throw himself into the sea to obtain relief or threaten to do so. And, of course, as is now well known, mental instability, amounting to delirium is one of the manifestations of severe cases of heatstroke, whether induced in or out of sunlight. According to the second, autotoxic, theory, the high temperature caused 'blood to become poisonous to the nerve cells', whilst the microbic theory attributed it to some micro-organism. This latter theory, however, *The Lancet* thundered, 'can hardly be sustained' and for the simple reason that the 'supposed microbe has not yet been seen.' The fourth – now disproved – theory, and the one that the leader backed, was the actinic theory which attributed heatstroke to the sun – hence the title of the leader.

This concept of sunstroke, as is discussed in the next chapter, died hard. Thus, in the notorious Mesopotamian campaign of the 1914–18 War, the experts could not clear themselves of the idea, the consulting physician to the Mesopotamian Expeditionary Force, stressing 'the necessity to wear a head protection – e.g. a topee', and urging that 'spinal pads 9 inches wide were necessary for the protection of the spinal cord from the sun's rays.' Even Sir Leonard Hill, the eminent physiologist, felt constrained to recommend 'a light sun helmet well ventilated and impermeable to sun rays.' But perhaps the most vivid picture of the state of affairs, and of medical thought, is that of the Earl of Carnarvon in his entertaining reminiscences, *No Regrets*.

> 'Some idea as to the stupefying effect of the heat at Basra may be judged from the fact that just before our arrival, the British Army lost 360 men by death from heatstroke. At one point during the height of the mid-day sun the wet and dry

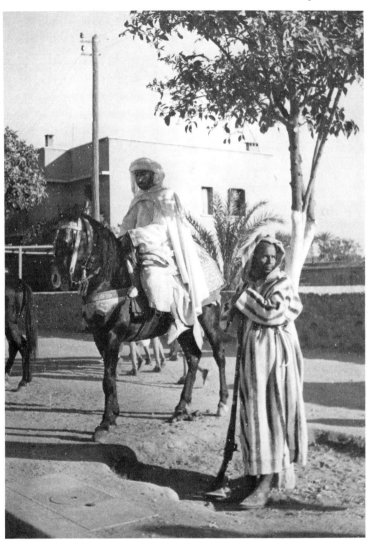

Moroccan Arabs.

bulbs on the barometers and thermometers were within 1 degree of coinciding. If they had done so, all human life would have become extinct because the temperature of the blood inside the body would have equalled that of the air outside. Fortunately our regiment was blessed with an absolutely first class medical officer, whose name was Captain Pettit. Later he was to win a M.C. In his rich Irish brogue he counselled everyone as follows. "There's only one hope for you, boys. I want each man to take off all his clothes and get inside his tent. Soak your towel, socks or anything else and lie down with them placed on your foreheads. Keep your heads moist and drink as much plain water as you want. In this way you should be all right. So lie down, don't move and stay calm".'

Perhaps not altogether the soundest of advice, especially in view of the poor protection from heat provided by tents. In the double ply E.P. tents then in use the temperature would often reach 135° to 140° F. (57° to 60° C.), and a little salt (sodium chloride) in the water would have been advisable. On the other hand, at least the Earl of Carnarvon obviously found the reassurance helpful and lived to tell the tale, and old soldiers will appreciate the point that, whereas the advice to the infantryman was for long 'keep your powder dry', the advice in 'Mespot' was 'keep your head moist'.

Even by the outbreak of the 1939–45 War ideas on the causation of heatstroke were still somewhat hazy, as exemplified in Peter Cochrane's *Charlie Company*: 'Eventually in the middle of August 1941, I got away, travelling down to Massawa to sail for Suez in a little steamer, all tattered red plush and no ventilation. It was crowded with South African soldiers, burly men oppressed by the heat; in Massawa it was well over 120° in the shade, and the Red Sea afforded no relief. The deck was packed with men kicking and floundering with heat stroke, and three of them died.' Research work, however, carried out during, and after, the War has clarified the issue. Not only do we know that it is caused by exposure to excessive heat, but, as one authority has put it, 'heatstroke is not a disease. It is a most unfortunate accident which is both foreseeable and preventable'. The effect of heat ranges from the relatively mild condition known as heat exhaustion to heatstroke itself, which a United States physician has described as 'a catastrophic disorder, characterised by hyperpyrexia (rectal temperature greater than 41.1°C. [106°F.]), delirium, coma and anidrosis [absence of sweating]'.

From all of which it is perfectly clear that hot climes play an important part in the maintenance of health. The essential basis of it all is that what is known as the core temperature of the body, that is the temperature usually ascertained in the rectum, must be maintained within a relatively narrow range, the upper limit being around 106° F. (42° C.). Beyond this, convulsions occur leading to death at 108° to 110° F. (42.6° to 43.7° C.). If consciousness is to be maintained, the core temperature must remain within 90° to 106° F. (32° to 42° C.), whilst functional efficiency is impaired if it moves beyond the range of 97° to 103° F. (36° to 48° C.).

To keep the temperature within these limits the body has an incredibly efficient compensatory system. The first line of defence is what is known as the vasomotor system. This is the system whereby the blood-vessels can dilate or constrict, that is, widen or narrow. In practice what this means is that, when exposed to heat, whether natural (e.g. the sun) or artificial (e.g. a furnace), and the temperature of the body begins to rise, a message is sent to a centre in that part of the brain known as the hypothalamus, in response to which a message is sent out which causes the blood-vessels of the skin to dilate. This immediately results in an increased volume of the blood passing through the skin and losing heat, as the external temperature is lower than that of the body. This cooled blood on its way back to the heart helps to keep the core temperature of the body down. It is this increased blood flow to the skin that makes it feel hot and become red, though, of course, reddening of the skin can also be caused by the ultra-violet radiation of the sun preliminary to tanning.

If this is not sufficient to keep the temperature of the body from rising, then the second, and really much more important, line of defence is called into action: namely, sweating. This again is a reflex action, induced through a centre in the brain. Once it has been initiated in this way, the amount of sweating is potentiated by the temperature of the hypothalamus. It is by evaporation of sweat that the body loses heat. This is why sweat dripping from the body is of little help in keeping the temperature down. It is only when it stays on the skin until it is evaporated that it induces the loss of heat from the body, for which it is intended.

There are more than two million sweat glands in the body. They are densest on the palms of the hands, the soles of the feet and the armpits, but these do not respond to heat; they are brought into action by mental and emotional stimuli, which explains why our hands start sweating when we are anxious – as when waiting for an examination or a critical interview. It is this sweating response to anxiety that is the rationale of the so-called 'lie detector' so beloved of the addicts of thrillers. In those parts of the body the density is around 2000 per square centimetre. Elsewhere they vary in density from 200 to 300 per square centimetre on the face and forehead to 80 to 200 on the limbs and trunk of the body. About half of the total sweat produced on a hot day comes from the skin on the trunk, a quarter from the lower limbs, and the rest from the upper limbs and head.

There are contradictory reports as to whether or not the coloured races have more sweat glands than the white races, but it seems to be agreed that they sweat more efficiently, as white people do when they become acclimatised to hot climates. On average they have a lower rate of sweating. Thus, as one observer has put it, 'at times when the white man has sweat pouring from his face and forehead, the brown man shows only a fine, velvet-like layer on his skin.'

On the other hand, there is impressive evidence of differences between the sexes. The sweating rate is lower in women, and they do not start sweating as quickly as men. Various factors are said to contribute to this state of affair. One is that women have a lower basal metabolic rate and therefore can maintain their temperature within normal limits at a higher environmental temperature than men. Another is that, in general, women have a thicker layer of subcutaneous fat (i.e. under the skin), and this helps to insulate the body against high external temperatures. It has also been suggested that for social reasons women probably prefer to avoid sweating more than men. In addition they usually wear lighter clothing, and in general take less part in athletic activities demanding a high level of energy expenditure. In the words of a Medical Research Council team that investigated this problem, it therefore follows that they 'exhibit the lower sweating capacity and higher sweating threshold which characteristise unacclimatized individuals.'

Several further points are worth noting, though briefly. One is that less heat can be lost by evaporation in hot humid weather than in hot dry weather, which explains why the former is so much more trying, and also dangerous from the point of view of developing heatstroke. Another is that adjustment, or acclimatisation to heat is much more difficult at the two extremes of life. This explains why old people, babies and young children are much more susceptible to heat. As a World Health Organisation report puts it: 'The physiological strains due to moderate and high levels of heat stress increase with age, mainly because of reduced cardiovascular capacity. The response of sweat glands to temperature changes becomes more sluggish as age increases, so that sweating becomes less effective as a mechanism for controlling body temperature.' In the case of babies the risks are increased by their greater turnover of water than adults, which means that, unless an adequate supply of water is maintained, they are liable to go downhill very quickly.

Sweat contains a relatively large amount of salt, or sodium chloride. This means that the profuse sweating that occurs in hot climes induces a large loss of salt from the body. If this is carried far enough it results in what are known as heat cramps, due to lack of the sodium ion. The drinking of large amounts of fluid to compensate for the amount lost in sweat exacerbates this shortage of sodium as more and more is lost in the sweat without any replacement. To compensate for this it is essential that those living in hot climes, especially if they are indulging in physical exertion, should take a daily increment of salt in their food and in their fluid intake. It is an interesting feature of the acclimatisation process to hot climates that the amount of salt in the sweat gradually falls.

In high temperatures the main strain falls on the heart and circulation, known as the cardiovascular system. This is why it is people with heart trouble who must be particularly careful about hot climes. To compensate for this extra strain and maintain an efficient circulation of blood – the *sine qua non* of healthy living – three main compensatory measures come into action. One is an increase in the maximum output of blood the heart can cope with. Another is an increase in the volume expelled by each beat of the heart, whilst the third is a diminution in the peak heart rate. By these means the healthy heart can cope with the increased demands of hot climes but, as will be obvious, these changes put increasing demands on the heart, which the damaged heart may not be able to meet, as is discussed in chapter 12.

Other compensatory measures are an increase in the volume of the sweat and a decrease in the amount of salt it contains. Men doing hard physical labour under hot conditions may sweat at a rate of as much as two litres an hour, and for periods of twenty-four hours there are records of up to twelve litres of sweat being produced. Once an individual becomes acclimatised to hot climes the daily loss of sweat tends to fall, probably as a result of increased metabolic efficiency. The accompanying diminished amount of salt, which results from the action of a hormone known as aldosterone, helps to ensure that the body is able to retain sufficient of the sodium ion in the body to maintain the delicate ionic equilibrium so essential to efficient functioning. One final, rather obvious, compensatory measure may be mentioned, and that is a decrease in the amount of urine that is passed.

This is not a medical textbook and therefore not the place to consider that 'catastrophic disorder', as heatstroke has been described, but there are lesser degrees of heat stress that are much more common, and should be recognised as a warning that the time has come to put the brake on. The least of these is a feeling of lassitude and irritability. Everything becomes an effort and everyone is an irritant. Whilst this is a state of affairs not unknown in temperate climes, where as often as not it is psychological in origin, in the tropics it is more likely to be of physical origin and due to lack of adequate acclimatisation. For long it was known as tropical neurasthenia, and there is undoubtedly a type of individual who fails dismally to come to terms with tropical life, no matter how well adjusted she (or he) may be physically. The remedy, if the cause is faulty acclimatisation, is to adhere more carefully to the rules of healthy living in the tropics: adequate ventilation indoors, correct clothing, an adequate intake of (non-alcoholic) fluid and of salt, and a modicum of physical exercise.

A slightly more distressing state of affairs, not uncommmon in hot climes, is to experience giddiness, sickness, general discomfort and acute physical fatigue, possibly accompanied by fainting. This is due to collapse of vasomotor control of the circulation, resulting in low blood pressure, so that the heart is unable to maintain an adequate circulation of blood. It is most likely to occur soon after entering a hot climate and is often provoked by taking too much physical exercise before first becoming acclimatised.

Anything like excessive exercise should be avoided on first entering a hot climate, and the amount of exercise should be gradually increased. This is particularly true for the middle-aged. The young can get away with a lot if basically they are physically fit, but age takes its toll, and the golden rule for those past their prime (which I refuse to define in precise terms) is to emulate Gilbert's mandarin: 'slow and stately, most sedately'.

Even for the young, however, there is a limit beyond which they cannot be stretched with safety. As a United States expert has commented: 'It is clear that fatal heatstroke can occur in perfectly healthy, highly acclimatised and physically conditioned individuals when the physical means to dissipate heat are exceeded by endogenous heat production.' He adds that 'in U.S.A. the majority of such cases occur in non-professional football players and military recruits. In the case of footballers many are young, highly competitive, inexperienced and over-enthusiastic, so do not pace themselves.' But the picture he paints is a disturbing one when he refers to 'certain practices in physical conditioning programmes that undoubtedly favour the propensity to incur heatstroke.'

'Flagrant among these', he notes, 'is the false notion that water deprivation accelerates acquisition of the conditioned state. To enforce this misconception, during football practice sessions, water may be provided only as a tepid, salted solution containing dissolved oatmeal in order to discourage its consumption. Another example is the provision of only salted water in canteens for soldiers in basic training . . . Ingestion of excessive sodium and insufficient water is a potentially lethal combination and undoubtedly accounts for cases of severe water-depletion heat exhaustion that culminates in severe heatstroke. Another potentially disastrous practice is based on the notion that strenuous exercise such as long-distance running in hot climes while clothed in impervious plastic sweat clothing will safely accelerate weight loss in overweight athletes.'

I know not how widespread such crude practices may be, but a similar warning comes from Tel-Aviv University in a report on thirty-six healthy young men who 'fell victims to heatstroke while engaged in strenuous physical exertion', eight of whom died as a result. The report ends with these somewhat astringent comments.

'The tragedy of heatstroke is that it so often strikes highly motivated young individuals, under the discipline of work, military training and sporting endeavour. Under other circumstances the same individuals would have rested when tired, drunk when thirsty, or remained at home when ill. It follows that the prevention of heatstroke requires adequate rest and hydration prior to physical exertion, as well as periods of rest during work when the individual can "cool off" and drink adequately. Such precautions should be implemented even in temperate zones during the hot summer months. In tropical zones physical exertion during the hottest hours should be avoided. These common-sense measures should not only prevent heatstroke, but also make for more efficient physical performance.'

No matter how man may abuse heat, as he abuses most things in his stupidity, many of us have to learn to live in hot climes, and indeed do so with considerable success. So much so that it has even been suggested that hot climes are best – even for the white races. First of all, however, what might be described as the more conventional view, as put forward in the *Annals of the New York Academy of Sciences*, may be summarised.

'It is apparent that Negroes do not do well in extreme cold and may not flourish at high altitudes. They seem to be well equipped, however, to deal with heat, at least of the moist tropical variety. Mongoloid people, on the other hand, seem best equipped to cope with the cold; it may not be a matter of sheer coincidence that the high altitude areas of the Himalayas and Andes are occupied by quasi-Mongoloid people. Mongoloids also thrive in the tropics of both hemispheres and as a whole seem to be the closest approach to an "all-purpose" man. Whites, who have pre-empted most of the best lands of temperate climate, do well in at least moderate cold and desert heat, but their history in the tropics leave them less than unqualified successes.'

The contrary view was presented in *Nature*, the doyen of scientific journals which has for long maintained the respect of international science.

'Man is best suited to the warm equable environment of a tropical forest, with its small diurnal variation in temperature and the protection it affords from heat gain from solar radiation during the day and heat loss by radiation to a clear sky at night . . . The critical temperature for man (25–27° C.) is at the upper range for tropical animals . . . European men previously adapted to life in temperate climes display after a period of some eighteen months' residence in Singapore, an ability to work in the heat that is markedly superior to that of similar men living in England, and equal to that possessed by the indigenous Malay, Chinese and Indian inhabitants . . . It is to be concluded therefore that a temperate clime does not represent the neutral conditions in which environmental stress is minimal and from which adaptation is possible both to hotter and to colder conditions in equal degree. On the contrary, man in a temperate clime is approaching the extreme range of adaptation to cooler conditions – i.e. maximal adaptation to cold.'

A stimulating and provocative thought in these days of *laissez-faire*, or permissiveness as it is currently known. A little more mental stimulus, and a little less transquillising, might well be what we all need today – even in considering climes that heal. Certainly in the cold London fog in which this chapter is being completed it is a pleasant thought that warms — metaphorically if not literally – the cockles of one's heart.

8

Hazards and benefits of sunshine

'Mad dogs and Englishmen go out in the mid-day sun', sang Noel
Coward but, until quite recently, the latter only with their heads
covered. Sunstroke was the dreaded penalty which the white man
paid for venturing into the tropical sun without his sun helmet or
topi. The respect, or rather fear, in which the tropical sun was held,
and the vulnerability of the human head as the assumed means
whereby sunstroke was induced, are admirably illustrated by two
excerpts from Dr Albert Schweitzer's *On The Edge of The Primeval
Forest*, published in 1922.

Describing his voyage out when he first went to French
Equatorial Africa, he writes: 'The day after we left Teneriffe the
troops were ordered to wear their sun helmets whenever they were
outside the saloon and cabins. This precaution struck me as
noticeable, because the weather was still cool and fresh, hardly
warmer than it is with us in June, but on the same day I got a
warning from an "old African", as I was enjoying the sight of the
sunset with nothing on my head. "From today onwards", he said,
"you must, even though the weather is not yet hot, regard the sun
as your worst enemy, and that whether it is rising, or high, in the
heavens, or setting, and whether the sky is cloudy or not. Why this
is so, and on what the sun's power depends, I cannot tell you, but
you may take it from me that people get dangerous sunstroke

before they get close to the equator, and that the apparently mild heat of the rising or setting sun is even more treacherous than the full glow of that fiery body at midday".'

The lesson was well taken, and soon after arrival at his destination he writes: 'I decided to promote to the rank of hospital the building which my predecessor in the house had used as a fowlhouse . . . It was, indeed, horribly close in the little windowless room, and the bad state of the roof made it necessary to wear my sunhelmet all day.' It was a subject about which he became quite obsessional, as indicated by the following comment: 'I was again called upon to go to N'Gomo. Mrs Faure had, without thinking, walked a few yards in the open without anything on her head and was now prostrate with severe fever and other threatening symptoms. Truly my fellow-traveller on the *Europe* was right when he said that the sun was our great enemy.'

And a decade later he still nursed this idée fixée, when he writes in *More From The Primeval Forest*: 'For a good many weeks after Whitsuntide I feel unwell . . . I have to drag myself to work and I am scarcely back from the hospital at midday and in the evening when I have to lie down. I cannot even manage to make out the order for necessary drugs and dressings. It is the roof of the hospital that is chiefly to blame for this. I had not noticed that it showed again a number of holes, and I no doubt got several slight sunstrokes.'

Dr Schweitzer may not have been as good a doctor as he was a theologian and organist, but the fearful respect in which he held the sun, and the dire necessity of protecting the head from its baneful influence were merely typical of contemporary thought. Yet as long ago as 1911 it had been shown experimentally that monkeys, with their bodies in the shade and only their heads unprotected, could be exposed to tropical sunshine for several days, from morning to afternoon, without any ill effect. One monkey had been exposed in this way to a total of fifty-four hours in twelve days, and, it was reported, 'the animal is still healthy and well.' Temperatures up to 116° F. (47° C.) were recorded in the hair of the head, but the rectal temperature never went above normal. What was entirely overlooked was that you do not get sunstroke in Alpine resorts, no matter how brilliant the sunshine. Today we realise that what the older generation called sunstroke was what we now know as heatstroke, and that the head is no more sensitive to heat than any other part of the body. The hazards of heat are discussed in the previous chapter. Here we are concerned with the direct results of the sun – baleful and benign – on the human body.

'Man must be in the light,' it has been said, 'the sun is necessary for life'. The important part of the solar spectrum, with which we shall be concerned in this chapter, is the ultra-violet radiation, which in moderation is beneficial, but in excess is harmful. This is a lesson that has penetrated the entire realm of Nature. Thus, desert plants are protected by hair, which scatters and absorbs the ultra-violet radiation. Animals, too, are supplied with hair or fur, with their protective action, while others, perhaps not so well protected, avoid excessive exposure by sleeping by day and working a night shift, by living largely in the shade, or by developing a pigmented skin. As a United States observer pointed out in the Philippine Islands some sixty years ago: 'The monkey, whose home is in the Tropics, withstands the sun less readily than any other animal I have observed, including even the white man. Of course, the monkey does not live in the fields; his home is in the forest, into which only a small proportion of the direct rays of the sun can enter. He instinctively avoids exposing himself to the sun for more than a few minutes.' He also drew attention to the fact that many a native of the tropics, 'even if otherwise nearly naked, often wears a large hat-like arrangement which shades not only his head but also his body.'

Man in his wellnigh hairless condition, apart from his head, is particularly vulnerable to the sun's radiation. One of his adaptations to overcome this handicap is his upright posture which, in the somewhat technical, but pleasingly concise, language of an expert, 'maximizes heat absorption at the end of the day and minimizes the area of direct insolation around noon. With the sun directly overhead the solar projection involves principally the head and shoulders. The head, of course, is well protected by the scattering and absorptive properties of the scalp hair.' Skin exposed to sunlight is protected by means of the brown pigment known as melanin.

The role of melanin in protecting man from ultra-violet radiation extends beyond the individual to racial groups. Almost all groups indigenous to the tropics have black skin. Moving polarwards there is a gradient through brown to the lighter skin of northern latitudes. According to the anthropologists, the light skin of the white races maximises the synthesis of vitamin D, while the dark skin of tropical races protects the skin from excessive ultra-violet radiation. A further evolutionary factor that has been mooted is that the lightly pigmented eyes that usually accompany a white skin – certainly in the Celtic races of the north – provided survival value advantages to their ancestors in low light levels, especially in the red light of dawn, sunset and firelight.

Before passing to a consideration of the effects of the sun, several interesting points call for attention. One is that the colour of the skin is a composite of four colours: brown, yellow, red and blue. The brown is that of the melanin pigment which is responsible for suntan. The yellow is that of pigments known as carotenoids which are contained in the food we eat (e.g. carrots), while the red and blue are contributed by the blood passing through the skin: the red of the oxygenated blood coming from the lungs, and the blue of the blood returning to the lungs, having disposed of its oxygen to the tissues of the body.

Whilst the tanning of the skin on exposure to the sun is due to its ultra-violet radiation, darkening of the skin can also be produced by hormones produced in the body. This is the cause of the darkening of the skin during pregnancy: around the nipples of the breasts, under the eyes and elsewhere. It is hormones, too, that are responsible for the seasonal change of colour of certain animals, such as the weasel, arctic fox and Greenland lemming. These hormonal changes, which are effected by light passing through the eyes to reach the pituitary gland, the master hormone-gland at the base of the brain, also affect the reproductive cycle so that during the winter these animals become 'reproductively quiescent'. To what extent hormones play a part in determining what has been described as constitutive skin colour is an open question still, but it has been suggested that they may be responsible for the diminution in the number of melanocytes (the cells that produce melanin) in the skin that occurs in old age.

Curiously enough, this hormonal aspect of sunlight is linked up with the public health problem of the 'windowless environment' of modern urban life. As a result of the widespread use of fluorescent lighting in schools, offices and factories today, a large proportion of the community spends a considerable number of working hours under what have been described as 'light spectra which differ considerably from those that characterise natural sunlight, and which are chosen by the lighting industry in accordance with the belief that the only significant effect of visible light on man was to enable him to perceive objects by their relative brightness' and which minimise the emission of ultra-violet radiation. Thus, the light intensity provided at eye level is usually less than 10 per cent of that present out of doors in the shade. 'The decision that this particular intensity was appropriate for indoor use', it has been said, 'seems to have been based upon economic and technological considerations rather than on any knowlege of man's biological needs', especially in view of the fact that 'considerable evidence is now available that environmental lighting, in the visible and near-ultra-violet ranges, does considerably more to man than to colour his skin or to provide the substrate for his vision.'

A United States observer has summed up the position: 'If a citizen of Boston lives in a conventionally lighted environment for sixteen hours per day, the total amount of visible light to which he is exposed is considerably less than would impinge upon him were he to spend a single hour each day out of doors.'

Whether or not there is any medical advantage in tanning the skin by exposure to sunshine is an open question apart from the production in the skin of vitamin D, which is essential for healthy living and the development of bone. This, of course, is why children deprived of sunlight develop rickets, characterised by bending and distortion of the bones of the body. A similar condition in adults is known as osteomalacia (literally, softening of the bones), most tragically seen in child-bearing women in whom it causes such distortion of the bones of the pelvis that birth *per vias naturales* is impossible, with resultant death of the unborn child unless skilled obstetric assistance is available. It is also the increasing heritage of the old folk in our midst, as a result of faulty diet and lack of sunshine, and resulting all too often in broken legs.

Lack of sunshine, it has hitherto been claimed, can in this respect be compensated for by taking vitamin D in the form of cod-liver oil or as tablets. According to Professor I. A. Magnus, however, in his monograph on *Dermatological Photobiology*, 'the generally held view that vitamin D requirements may be adequately or conveniently covered by a "normal" diet or oral medication may have to be revised if it can be confirmed that these requirements are more efficiently met, as is suspected, by skin irradiation, solar or artificial.'

There is also some evidence of its being of value in the treatment of that most chronic of skin conditions: psoriasis. Over the years practically everything in turn has been recommended to the victims of this distressing, scale-like affliction of the skin, from tar to the waters of the Dead Sea. Recently there has been a rapid development in the world-wide use of a combination of long-wave ultra-violet radiation and a drug known as methoxsalen. Known as PUVA, this combined therapy is currently being evaluated at various centres in the United Kingdom, from which promising preliminary results are being reported. In the past ultra-violet radiation has proved of value in the treatment of lupus vulgaris, or tuberculosis of the skin, a form of treatment for the introduction of which the distinguished Danish doctor, Niels

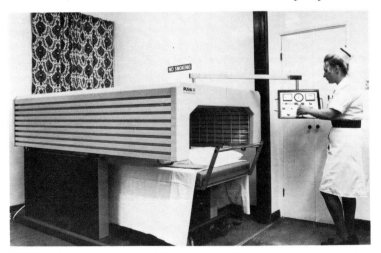

PUVA unit at the Institute of Dermatology, London: patients suffering from psoriasis receive alternate-day administration of methoxsalen combined with exposure to high-intensity long-wavelength ultra-violet (UVA) irradiation.

Finsen, was awarded the Nobel Prize for medicine in 1903, and of other forms of non-pulmonary tuberculosis. Today, however, the introduction of streptomycin and other anti-tuberculosis drugs has rendered this use of ultra-violet radiation redundant.

Whether sunlight, or phototherapy as it is technically known, has any further action is once again the sixty-four thousand dollar question. The cult of the sun has always been with us since the days of the ancient Greeks, if not earlier, and its advocates today are just as enthusiastic about the wonderful effect it has. For them it is the modern elixir of life, keeping them fit and giving them a zest for life unobtainable in any other way. That these sun-tanned members of the community feel better there can be no doubt, but how much of this improvement is psychological? Again and again, just as doctors are becoming convinced that the benefit is psychological, further evidence is forthcoming that suggests that there is more to it than this. And at the moment we are in one of these phases.

Much of this new work comes from Germany and Russia, and seems to show that in normal human subjects simple tasks requiring physical exertion are performed more efficiently after irradiation with ultra-violet light, and that such irradiation during the winter increases resistance to infection. So impressed are the Russians with this evidence that they have made ultra-violet therapy compulsory for coal-miners. It is difficult not to be impressed, though not necessarily convinced, by this evidence. Certainly it should not be turned down too peremptorily, and there will be many who will agree with the opinion expressed in *Sunlight and Man*, the proceedings of the 1972 International Conference on Photosensitization, which was published in 1974 and quickly earned a reputation as a goldmine for the seeker after knowledge on the subject.

> 'Much of the literature on phototherapy says that one of the most common indications was "asthenia". With success in the treatment of some common infections and reduction in some acute infections we cannot help but wonder whether ultra-violet radiation to the skin aids the body's immune systems in some way. A source of uncertainty in many of the older studies is the possibility that the patients may have had deficiency of vitamin D. However, I believe the time is ripe to reopen many of the avenues of investigation in both phototherapy and immunology [the study of the defence mechanism of the body against infection] that were delayed by the antibiotic era. Perhaps this will help us understand why we like sunshine and dislike "dreary" days.'

As a possibly plebeian postscript to this consideration of the benefits, and possible benefits, of ultra-violet radiation may be added a note to the effect that many still find this a useful method of preventing chilblains. In the cautious words of *Black's Medical*

Dictionary: 'Carefully controlled irradiation with ultra-violet light from a carbon-arc lamp is often beneficial.'

Such are the benefits of sunlight. The hazards are threefold. The first is the commonplace sunburn, which may vary from a temporary sense of discomfort to a severe systemic disturbance, with severe blistering of the skin, that has ruined many a holiday. In the vast majority of cases it can be avoided if one elementary rule is observed, and a few elementary facts are remembered. Never over-expose yourself to sunlight. This involves gradual initiation to sunbathing, starting off with only a few minutes exposure at the beginning of the season or holiday, and gradually lengthening this according to the reaction of the skin. As Professor Magnus has said: 'Sunburn can be prevented. Once it has been provoked, standard creams and lotions usually suffice.'

Among the facts to be remembered the elementary one is that fair complexioned people are more liable to sunburn than dark complexioned people, but dark hair is not necessarily a guarantee against it. There is a seasonal variation in sensitivity to ultra-violet radiation. In Northern Europe sensitivity decreases during late spring and early summer, to increase again in the autumn. This seasonal difference is related to a thickening of the skin and an increased production of melanin. The intensity of the sunburn range of ultra-violet radiation varies with the position of the sun, being maximal at noon, and reduced by three-quarters of its strength by late afternoon. Sunburn becomes impossible with complete cloud cover, but on a hazy day with cloud it is possible to receive up to 80 per cent of the amount of ultra-violet radiation present on a bright day without clouds. The risk of over-exposure in these circumstances, it has been pointed out, 'is increased because the clouds filter the infra-red radiation that normally causes the sensation of heat that acts as a danger signal.'

Shade will not necessarily prevent sunburn. Scattering of ultra-violet radiation from the sky may be sufficiently strong to induce sunburn, which may then occur when in the shade, as, for instance, sitting under a parasol. Incidentally, in this context, it should be remembered that sand reflects ultra-violet radiation. Hence, as it has been put, 'a person can be burned by both radiation from the sky and reflection from the sand.'

Water is a poor reflector of ultra-violet radiation, but snow is an excellent reflector. As the ultra-violet spectrum of sunlight increases with height, being, for example, 20 per cent greater at 5000 feet (1500 metres) than at sea level, this explains why the wearing of ultra-violet-proof goggles is essential at snow-bound heights. If not worn, the painful condition known as snow blindness is easily induced.

Another point to be borne in mind, particularly amid the snow, is that a wind can enhance the effect of the sun, as Joseph Chamberlain found to his cost. In a letter to his mother from Moulanvers, near Chamonix, in August 1857, he wrote: 'I am brown as mahogany nearly but am at present sadly disfigured by very bad lips made sore by the cold wind.' Three years later, according to Denis Judd in *Radical Joe*, 'he writes from Zermatt, complaining that his face and lips are swollen by the cold winds and adding a wry postscript: "I forgot to say that I have made a valuable correction to a commonly received scientific statement, that which says that the skin comes off once in seven years. No such thing! The skin of the face and neck comes off in seven days like a very bad thin brown paper in strips an inch long and half an inch broad. The new skin is very red and tender and is chosen as a delightful recreation ground for juvenile flies".'

So-called advances in medicine have made their contribution to the problems of sunburn. Quite a number of the much-vaunted drugs that the pharmaceutical industry, with the all too willing cooperation of the medical profession, have foisted on the public are liable to produce a condition known as photosensitivity, which renders the skin more subject to sunburn. Anyone taking drugs therefore, who is proposing to take a sunshine holiday, or to indulge in sunbathing in his garden, should consult his family doctor to make sure that he is not taking a drug that might cause photosensitivity. Equally important is it to remember that certain cosmetics may induce photosensitivity. In this respect, advice should be sought from a doctor or from an experienced cosmetician, taking care not to be misled by the conception that the more expensive the cosmetic the less likely is it to produce this distressing sensitivity of the skin to sunlight.

Finally, it is useful to know that moving about reduces the risk of sunburn. It is the recumbent sunbather who is asking for trouble – and gets it as often as not.

The most important hazard of sunlight is cancer of the skin, due to over-exposure to a certain range of the ultra-violet rays of the sun. This is rare among pigmented races, and is most liable to occur in those of Celtic stock with fair complexions and blue eyes who tan poorly, and have a history of repeated sunburn. In the words of a Glasgow dermatologist; 'The fair-skinned Celtic people can suffer disastrous long-term effects from exposure to tropical sun, in the form of multiple skin cancer, and it is desirable that this fact should be as widely known in the lands of their birth as it is in the sunny countries to which they often emigrate; and that it should be translated into prophylactic advice, such as: *Do not go and live in the tropics if you have a fair skin that burns easily in the sun.* It is important to realize that the damage accumulates throughout life, and that it becomes visible insidiously. The level of solar radiation obtaining in Scotland is sufficient to induce similar changes, but on a much smaller scale, especially in people who have lived out of doors.' The italics are his, not mine.

Its incidence ranges from about 380 per 100 000 among white Australians to around 1.7 per 100 000 among Bantus in South Africa. The high incidence in Australia is, of course, due to the predominantly white population, many of whom live, and have open-air jobs, in areas with a superfluity of sunshine such as pertains in the north of the continent. The Australian craze for sunbathing does nothing to lower its incidence. In Britain it is a relatively remote hazard.

A more common hazard that need be mentioned is a chronic degenerative condition of the skin which has been epitomised by

Professor Magnus as: increased dryness and cracking of the skin; increased patchy pigmentation of the skin; atrophy and decreased elasticity of the skin; localised thickening of the outer layer of the skin; a tendency to bleed from the small blood-vessels of the skin, producing what are known as ecchymoses. These changes, he notes, 'may be difficult to separate from what is commonly put down to "natural" ageing, if indeed they can be distinguished at all.' 'Ultra-violet radiation', he adds, 'may merely be an accelerator of senescence.' Which, curiously enough, was the view of our Victorian grandmothers who refused to go out in the mid-day sun, or indeed any sun, without wide-brimmed hat and parasol, preferring to maintain the youthful beauty of their skin as long as possible, rather than bring on the ravages of old age sooner than necessary by exposing their skin to its devastating rays.

A final hazard of sunshine that may be mentioned is acne, or at least what the experts call acneiform reactions. This is most likely to occur after prolonged sunbathing, and is being increasingly seen by doctors in Britain in patients returning from a Mediterranean holiday – so much so that it is now commonly known as Majorca acne: an unpleasant price to pay for indiscriminate sunbathing. The curious anomaly here is that acne, as its victims know, usually improves during the summer, and it has always been thought that this was due to the extra sunshine. The probable explanation for this apparent anomaly is that the excessive sweating induced by over-indulgence in sunbathing induces the acneiform eruption.

In Northern Australia these degenerative changes in the skin may be found within the second decade of life, but in Britain they are rare except late in life in outdoor workers. It will be interesting to note in the future whether the current craze for sunbathing changes the British picture.

9

Hazards of man-made climes

Where do we go from here? Such is the question many are asking, but few are answering. Those who do answer tend to be the more hysterical in our midst and unfortunately these include not a few scientists who, as a genus, ought to know better. All too often, however, once they leave their bench and lift their eyes from their electronic microscopes, they lose all sense of balance, and panic. They insist on a physical explanation of the universe, including man, failing to realise that man is spirit as well as body. Lacking any faith, except on occasion a curious fantasy called humanism, they can see no end for man except self-destruction.

It is this lack of balance, due largely to a lack of religious faith, that is at the basis of so much of the nonsense talked about conservation. What is proposed in this chapter is merely to pick out some of the more important aspects of the problem in relation to climate. But perhaps the background can best be sketched in by a quotation from an article by Professor T. J. Chandler, the Professor of Geography in Manchester University.

'It took several hundred thousand years to reach the first billion human beings, around 1800, but only 130 years more were needed to add the second billion, and less than thirty years for the third by around 1960. Today we are two-thirds of the way to the fourth billion and the expectation is that well over two billions more will be added in the last quarter of the century. Such enormous increases of population cannot but extend and intensify climatological changes in the lower 600 metres or so of the atmosphere known as the planetary boundary layer and possibly, directly or indirectly, of the atmosphere as a whole. This is because the properties of the atmosphere are closely controlled by physical and chemical exchanges at the earth–air interface and these are a function of surface conditions such as the shape and surface cover of the land which will be increasingly changed as populations grow. In draining the marsh, clearing the woods, cultivating the fields, flooding the valleys and building towns man has inadvertently changed the thermal, hydrological and roughness parameters of the earth's surface and the chemical composition of the air. The intensity of the meteorological consequences will depend on a number of factors.'

One of the oldest problems in this sphere is that of atmospheric pollution arising from our use of natural resources as a source of energy. As long ago as the Roman Empire the Roman patricians were complaining about the soot that soiled their togas, and Seneca waxed eloquent in his denunciation of 'the heavy air of Rome and the stench of its smoky chimneys.' Medieval London was equally cursed by the smoke-polluted atmosphere, especially when the soft coal was brought in from Newcastle. As soon as records began to be kept it became evident that fog was responsible for a heavy loss of life from chronic bronchitis and heart failure every year, and its more virulent successor, smog, carried on and enhanced this dire effect on the pulmonary and cardiac cripples in our midst.

But this problem is not just confined to western civilisation. India has its pollution problem due to domestic fires. All over India the poor use cow dung cakes as fuel, and these produce considerable pollution of the atmosphere in the ill-ventilated huts in winter time. So much so that the high prevalence among young women in central India of the form of heart disease known as cor pulmonale is believed to be the result of exposure to these fumes. To cope with this problem and reduce the hazard to health, 'cow dung gas' – that is, cooking gas obtained by incineration of cow dung – is being introduced. This is comparable to commercial gas and is used in the same way, but produces much less pollution than the cow dung cakes. In addition, in rural India health programmes now include the popularisation of smokeless fires for cooking (chulas) which can be easily made from simple materials and which prevent the inhalation of smoke while working over them.

Much more worrying is what is known as the 'greenhouse effect' of carbon dioxide. According to a report issued by the U.S. National Academy of Sciences in 1977, if the use of fossil fuels, such as coal and oil, continues to increase at present rates, the average global temperature could rise by around 6° C. over the next two centuries. This is because carbon dioxide produced when coal and oil are burnt absorbs the heat radiated from the earth's surface. In other words it acts like the glass of a greenhouse, entrapping the sun's heat: hence the 'greenhouse effect'. It is estimated that the concentration of carbon dioxide in the atmosphere has increased 11 to 13 per cent from the beginning of the industrial revolution to today, that it may be increased by 25 per cent by the turn of the century, doubled by 2050 and increased four to eight times in two hundred years if the use of fossil fuels continues to increase.

Among the 'adverse, perhaps catastrophic' effects that could arise from this rise of temperature would be rises of sea levels of as much as 16 feet (5 metres) that would inundate capitals such as London and New York. The North American corn-belt would be pushed northwards off the productive soils of the middle west on to the poorer Canadian soils. In addition the warming of the surface layers of the oceans would reduce the natural vertical circulation, thereby reducing the biological productivity of the oceans by depressing the circulation of nutrients.

And so the grim list continues. Admittedly, as the experts on the committee are the first to admit, much is hypothesis, but it is scientifically sound hypothesis and at least justifies careful consideration of how the use of fossil fuels can be reduced. Just to complicate the issue, it would appear that the accelerated rate of deforestation of the world is accentuating the problem. Hitherto there has been the consoling knowledge that some part at least of this excess carbon dioxide was mopped up by the forests of the world. But it now appears that not only is this mopping up action being lost, but the amount of carbon dioxide being pumped into the atmosphere annually from fossil fuels may be equalled by that released from forests felled either directly for firewood or for agricultural clearance. Again much is hypothesis but, without being in the least alarmist, obviously, if he is to survive, mankind will need to take a long, keen look at where his race for 'worldly goods' is taking him.

An excess of ozone is another man-made climatic hazard, as was exemplified in the south-east of England during the 1976 heat wave, when for more than a week the amount of ozone far exceeded the safe limit. Normally the level of ozone in the atmosphere is around 30 parts per billion, and in industry the recommended safe upper limit is 80 parts per billion. During the 1976 heat wave the concentration in south-east England reached 250 parts per billion.

The cause of this excess atmospheric ozone is nitrogen oxide, the main source of which is the internal combustion engine, but other forms of industrial combustion can produce it. Normally much of this ozone is removed by natural methods but under anticyclonic conditions the accompanying inversions, as they are known, trap the ozone at night and the following day it is released and returned to earth. For some years it has been realised that pollution originating thousands of miles away in northern Europe can produce high ozone levels in England. This was what happened in July 1976 when the source was tracked down to Poland. The main health hazard of excess ozone is as a lung irritant, and it is therefore a particular hazard for those with asthma or chronic bronchitis.

But it is not only in excess that ozone can be a danger to health. Lack of it can be hazardous. This is because in the stratosphere, that dark blue layer of the atmosphere that surrounds us some five miles up and stretching outwards for around thirty miles, is composed of ozone. This layer of ozone cuts out a certain amount of the ultra-violet light from the sun and thereby protects us from excessive exposure. If it were not for this protective action of ozone in the stratosphere, not only would we tan much more easily (which might please the sunbathers), it would also expose us to the hazards of too much ultra-violet radiation, which include cancer of the skin.

The potential man-made climatic hazard here is the increasing use of domestic, cosmetic and gardening aerosols. What the sum total of all these come to now reaches astronomical figures: 6 billion a year in U.S.A. and around 500 million in the United Kingdom are typical of the figures being bandied about. The link-up between aerosols and ozone is the propellant in the former which belongs to a group of substances known as chlorofluoro-carbons. So stable are these that when released into the atmosphere they penetrate to the stratosphere. There they are finally decomposed by the intense ultra-violet radiation they encounter there. Unfortunately, this decomposition process releases chlorine atoms which link up with ozone and destroy it. In 1972 it was calculated that 'fluorocarbons are intentionally and accidentally vented to the atmosphere worldwide at a rate approaching 1 billion pounds a year.' If this rate is maintained it is estimated that the ozone content of the stratosphere will fall by around seven per cent.

How true a bill this is is still not quite clear, but the manu-facturers are taking avoiding action and finding substitutes for chlorofluorocarbons, so that there is probably little to worry about. On the other hand, it is but another illustration of the harm man may do by interfering with the atmosphere in which we live, move and have our being.

Lead is another much discussed man-made climatic hazard.

Currently the two main sources of lead as a health hazard – apart from certain industrial processes in which there is adequate legislation to safeguard the health of employees – are petrol and water. According to one committee member of the Campaign Against Lead in Petrol, 'no-one disputes that about 75 per cent of the lead in petrol ends up in the air as a fine aerosol, or that vehicle exhausts account for more than 90 per cent of lead in the air in cities. Lead also accumulates in the environment.' 'What is in dispute,' it is added, 'is the contribution of airborne lead to total body lead burdens, and whether these burdens are approaching (or have exceeded) safety limits.' Whatever the outcome of the current controversy, we in Britain are certainly lagging behind other countries. Thus, the British permitted maximum of 0.5 gramme of lead per litre of petrol compares with 0.15 in Germany. In the U.S.A. lead-free petrol is available at all but the smallest filling stations, and the average lead content of petrol containing it is to be reduced to 0.13 gramme by 1979. Japan has virtually banned lead entirely from petrol, whilst in the U.S.S.R. lead was eliminated from all petrol sold in cities in 1959.

We are equally lagging in our control of lead in drinking water, and it is claimed that the drinking water of around two million homes in Britain contains more lead than is allowed by E.E.C. standards, whilst in 800 000 houses it exceeds the World Health Organization standard which is twice as lax as that of the E.E.C. As in the case of petrol the experts tend to differ, and there is little doubt that the anti-lead protagonists are overplaying their hand. Conversely, however, we do know that lead is a definite health hazard, and it would seem to be commonsense, apart from any humanitarian motives, to reduce our exposure to toxic levels of lead to a minimum. In the case of petrol, why not lead-free petrol even though this might add, as has been estimated, 1 to 2 p. per gallon to the cost? Alternatively, why not insist on the manufacturers producing cars with medium compression-ratio engines to allow them to run on 91–92 octane fuel, which needs no lead? In the case of drinking water the obvious solution is gradually to eradicate all lead piping and tanks, starting off with those soft-water areas of country in which such pipes are most likely to lead to contamination in this way. As it is estimated that around ten million houses would be involved in this process at an estimated cost of £1000 million, obviously the elimination process must be a slow one. There is certainly no indication for any panic action.

Finally we come to something approaching science fiction. In 1977, *New Scientist* published an article entitled 'If tube trains affect trees, what do they do to us?', in the course of which it stated: 'Underground trains in San Francisco generate magnetic fields that are a thousand times stronger than the natural background. They are so strong that they set up measurable electric currents in trees.' This was based on a report from Stanford Radioscience Laboratory, according to which the influence on trees is so strong that it can be easily shown by hammering two nails one centimetre in a tree, one millimetre apart vertically, and linked to a voltmeter. The author's contention is that there must be a similar effect on people, and he is quoted as saying: 'The human body is an electrically conducting fluid – just a big sac of salty water. A fluctuating magnetic field in a conducting fluid sets up electric currents.' In addition, he rightly notes, cells have their own electrical field which could be affected by a varying electro-magnetic field.

All too often we find that the science fiction of today is the science fact of tomorrow. Is this a case in point? Is there a danger, as *New Scientist* suggests, that 'the large electromagnetic fields now being added to our environment may generate currents in the body which have long-term disruptive effects'? As the Stanhope author comments: 'No-one monitors our total exposure to electromagnetic fields (of all frequencies) and it is conceivable that the San Francisco signals, though probably harmless themselves, may increase the possibility of harm from other electromagnetic signals.' The risk may be remote, but it is certainly one that should be investigated. There is an old Scottish saying that 'mony a pickle maks a muckle', and there may well be a cumulative effect as suggested that in time might have a deleterious effect on the health of the community.

Typical of the 'mony pickles' is the electrostatic effects produced by the man-made fibres we are using to an ever-increasing extent. As one Danish investigator has put it: 'The wide application in modern buildings of materials and furniture with low conductivity and the use of synthetic fibres in furniture, textiles and clothes have resulted in man often finding himself in electrical fields in the course of everyday life.' To what extent are these electrical fields being modified, and to what extent are these modifications harmful, harmless, or even possibly beneficial? Certainly the days of 'magnetism' are returning if in a more scientific garb. Was there possibly something in the teaching and practice of mesmerism – apart from quackery or hypnotism? It all opens up an intriguing vista if only the younger generation will have the courage to take it up as a serious scientific problem.

10

The microclimate of the bedroom

Considering the fact that most of us spend around a third of our lives in bed, it is interesting how relatively little attention is given to the climate of the bedroom. All too often it is the coldest part of a British home in winter even in these days of central heating. Before the central-heating era going to bed in the average middle-class house could only be described as a purgatorial experience. In the language of one of our United States cousins what was forgotten was that 'the bed constitutes an escape from uncomfortable environmental conditions. It is an early invention of man to control his atmospheric surroundings. Even more than the room, it permits segregation of the body from adverse exposure to cooling influences.'

The ideal to be aimed at for comfort is a warm bed in a cool room. The temperature of the bedroom, it has been said, is 'a matter of taste, cost and what is available.' The coolness, of course, at least in winter in so-called temperate climates, refers to the temperature after the occupants are in bed. Apart from the young, few things are more soothing and conducive to sleep than a warm bedroom in which to get into bed. One recommendation is a temperature of 66° F. (19° C.) for young healthy persons and 75° F. (24° C.) for old people. According to one United States observer the 'comfortable range' is 68° to 71° F. (20° to 22° C.). This is more or less in accordance with current British views, expressed by one commentator as: 'Where English people can afford the cost of a comfortable bedroom they are willing to accept temperatures of even up to 70° F. (21° C.), above which it is deemed to be overwarm.' On the other hand, a perpetual temperature of this level throughout the whole night would probably be too high for comfort for many, and not the least of the advantages of central heating is that the temperature can be allowed to drop during the night and then raised before the time for getting up arrives.

'Stuffiness' must certainly be avoided. It is not only one of the antidotes to sound sleep; it is also liable to produce that awakening 'thick head' that is the worst possible start for the new day. It is not only the 'fresh air fiends' who derive pleasure from lying in a comfortably warm bed and feeling a cool, or even cold, breeze playing on the face from an open window in mid-winter. Incidentally, a practical point to be borne in mind is that bedrooms with open windows at night never reach the minimum temperature out of doors. Whilst hitherto the implied emphasis has been on winter conditions, the same principles apply in the summer. In hot weather the bedroom must be adequately ventilated, and in hot climes, if it is not air-conditioned, then air movement must be stimulated by means of a fan. In such climes, too, the bedroom windows must be shaded by blinds (venetian or otherwise) and sunshades during the heat of the day so as to keep the temperature of the bedroom down to a minimum. A diurnally sun-baked tropical bedroom will never be a comfortable nocturnal place of rest.

In considering the bed in wintry conditions such as we have in this country, several points must be borne in mind. One is that the temperature of the body falls during the night, but that of the skin tends to rise. This means that, unless the temperature in the bed is kept at a reasonable level, there will be an excessive loss of heat from the body, with a corresponding lowering of the body temperature. Opinions differ as to what is the ideal temperature under the bedclothes, but most people are comfortable in bed if this is around 89° to 90° F. (31° to 32° C.). In one investigation, in which the morning bedroom temperature was 54° F. (12.2° C.), the air temperature in a single bed was 77.4° F. (22.2° C.), while in 70 out of 100 observations the morning bed temperature was above 87° F. (30° C.).

The second point to be borne in mind is that the bed temperature is predominantly dependent on its initial temperature when it is first occupied. Thus, in one experiment it was found that when the bed temperature when first occupied was 60° F. (16° C.) on average it duly rose to 84° F. (29° C.), whereas when the initial temperature was 70° F. (21° C.) the maximum attained was around 91° F. (33° C.). Equally relevant is the fact that this means in practice that the rise to a comfortable temperature takes longer. In other words, our parents and theirs were right and the first essential of a comfortable night is a bed-warmer in some form or other.

Few things are more conducive to insomnia than cold feet, and the commonest cause of cold feet is the completely avoidable cold bed. Today the electric blanket has simplified the matter still further. Apart from anything else it has the practical advantage of spreading the heat more uniformly throughout the bed than a hot water bottle. On the other hand it cannot be cuddled, which is such a solace to many. A word of warning, however, should be interpolated here to the effect that the blanket should always be switched off before going to sleep, unless it is a low-wattage one. As an adjunct to a warm bed the old-fashioned bed-socks have a lot to be said in their favour.

Night clothes are a fairly recent innovation, people in the old days going to bed in their underwear or in the nude. Today they are the rule, except among the more exotic, who like to be different and are following the craze of going to bed in what they euphemistically describe as their 'birthday suit'. Whether pyjamas or a nightshirt be worn is a matter of taste, as is the material of which these are made. As Dr E. T. Renbourn has soundly put it in *Materials and Clothing in Health and Disease*: 'Since air, particularly that near the skin, is the essential factor governing body warmth, it is a wise belief that most non-prejudiced people will be just as warm in a fine, silk (or synthetic) fabric as they would be in a wool or raised cotton garment of greater thickness.' What is important to bear in mind, particularly for children and old folk, is that the material must be non-inflammable.

The same open attitude must be adopted towards the material of which sheets are made. Some prefer the luxurious cool sensation of linen, but it is merely an aesthetic advantage. Some prefer the apparent warmth of flannelette sheets, but this again is illusory so far as thermal insulation and heat retention are concerned, and their use should certainly not be encouraged for old folk who smoke in bed, because of the fire risk. The only objection to nylon sheets, and again it is of no great practical import, is the static electricity which they may generate, especially in the dry state induced by the electric blanket. There is, of course, no health reason for sheets, except that they help to keep the blankets clean.

The traditional woollen blanket still rules the bedroom roost. What tends to be forgotten is that this reputation for warmth is largely dependent upon the air entrapped in their interstices and, when several are used, between each blanket. This was the explanation of an interesting experiment in which it was shown that there is relatively little difference between two or three blankets from the point of view of warmth. The weight of the extra blanket cuts down the air space between the layers, thereby diminishing their powers of insulation. For those who dislike the weight of the woollen blanket there is now a wide range of lightweight synthetic blankets and cellular blankets.

Apart from lightness there is nothing to be said medically for the continental eider-down or feather-bed covering. They are perfectly efficient from the warmth point of view, but require considerable experience to prevent their being on the floor as often as on the sleeper. For those who like novelty and lightness, however, and are reasonably quiet sleepers, there is nothing against them.

Three final short points, or quickies, as Gilbert Harding used to call them on a one-time popular B.B.C. radio programme, may be made. The first is that where healthy adults are concerned the number of pillows is a matter of taste. Some prefer to be flat with one pillow. Others sleep better if propped up with two or even three pillows. Babies, of course, should not be given a pillow at all. The second is that asthmatic subjects should pay particular attention to their bedding lest this be the source of the cause of their attacks. The third is that the problem of the aged has only been referred to in passing. Fuller consideration of their important needs in this respect will be found in chapter 19.

I I

Climate and clothes

'The suitability of the clothing is of the greatest importance not only to the comfort but the efficiency of man as a working machine.' So wrote Sir Leonard Hill but, fortunately or otherwise – depending largely upon whether the problem is approached from the aesthetic or practical angle – this utilitarian aspect of clothes has all too often been overlooked. As Sir Leonard himself pointed out: 'Clothes protect us from the rubbing and tearing, the wetting and corroding action of the world. They afford means of ornament and sexual attraction, the decent privacy of sex, the notation of rank, occupation, and culture, and the means of imposture and exhibition of vanity and arrogance.' All of which was put rather more grandiloquently some eighty years earlier by Thomas Carlyle in *Sartor Resartus* (The Tailor Reclothed);

> 'Men's earthly interests are all hooked and buttoned up and held together by clothing. Clothes, too, which began in the foolishest love of ornament, what have they not become? Increased security and pleasurable heat soon follow, but what of these? Shame, divine shame, arose there mysteriously under the clothes . . . a mystic grove-encircled shrine for the Holy in man. Clothes gave us individuality, distinction, social polity; clothes have made men of us, they are threatening to make clothes screens of us.'

108

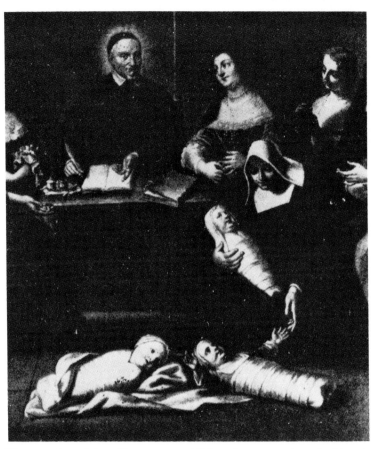

The practice of bundling young children into excessive clothing is centuries old. This painting was found in a Paris orphanage, but swaddling clothes were in common use 2000 years ago.

Certainly more nonsense has been talked about clothes – by fashion experts, advertisers, manufacturers, doctors and humanity in general alike – than on any other subject under the sun. Fortunes are made and lost by the manufacturers of man-made fibres – in 1977 the European man-made fibres industry lost £500 million. Men and women wear the most unsuitable clothes, inflicting on themselves untold misery and often health hazards, and at the same time spend sums of money on their clothes that they can ill afford. Today, perhaps, people are dressing more sensibly, but there is still much ignorance on the subject, or, alternatively, a persisting tendency to ignore the advice that is now freely available, much of which, incidentally, is based on information acquired as a result of careful research carried out during the 1939–45 War to find the best way of clothing our troops to allow them to face the hazards of fighting in cold and tropical climes.

For centuries, it has been said, the skin has been overburdened by an excess of clothing, the most flagrant example of which is the tendency still for many mothers to bundle up their children in excessive clothing. As has been pointed out, 'this encumbers the child so much that he cannot exercise normally and so becomes inactive, which lowers his metabolic heat production and so he becomes cold.' This, of course, is a remnant of the ancient custom of wrapping a babe in swaddling clothes, a practice probably initiated with the aim of ensuring that the limbs grew straight, although Soranus (A.D. 98–138), who has been described as the greatest gynaecologist and obstetrician of antiquity, recommended the procedure because the Roman baby became easily chilled because of the cold water which flowed beneath the city. That this habit of overclothing died hard is exemplified by the fact that as late as 1920 it was reported in the *Proceedings of the Institute of Hygiene* that children in elementary schools were wearing as many as thirteen different articles of clothing.

The ideal to be borne in mind is that the minimum of clothing should be worn consistent with reasonable comfort: an ideal going back at least to the days of Aristotle, according to whom, 'to accustom children to cold from their earliest years is an excellent practice which greatly conduces to health.' Some two millenia later the same point of view was being put forward by a Scottish general practitioner: 'The longer I work among people the more I find cases of individuals who habitually go with little clothing and still show the greatest immunity to those diseases commonly attributed to the influence of cold. I am becoming more and more convinced that a great deal more harm comes from overheating the body than is ever due to the influence of natural cold.'

A view shared by Almond, the famous headmaster of Loretto School, where until quite recent years the official school uniform was based on the wearing of shorts. To Almond fresh air and exercise were the two secrets of healthy living. One of his famous aphorisms was: 'I would consider the Chinese punishment of depriving of sleep as less dangerous than the depriving of exercise. It would be much better to put a boy on bread and water than do that.' And not only did he insist on shorts, he would never allow his boys to wear anything at all tight round the neck, realising, as Sir Leonard Hill put it, that 'the open neck acts as a flue for the escape of body heat, and the close collars worn by men are disadvantageous compared to the free opening which women indulge in to display their charms.'

The problem is to determine what is the optimal temperature, or at least the lowest temperature which can be tolerated with comfort. As has been pointed out: 'Primitive man can exist in the nude, without marked discomfort, at temperatures out-of-doors down to almost freezing point, with either the protection of a small fire or a small fur windbreak round one shoulder. This is exemplified by the Australian Aborigines of today who are exposed to the cold nights of the desert, and by the former inhabitants of Tierra del Fuego at the tip of the South American hemisphere who were exposed to the driving snow.' Nearer home, it was not so long ago – and, indeed, for all I know, unless they have joined a trade union, may still be the case – that artists' models thought nothing of sitting for several hours in the nude at temperatures that seldom, if ever, rose above 59° F. (15° C.), and showed no sign of distress or shivering.

According to Sir Leonard Hill,

'A civilized man when naked finds exposure to still air at 35° to 37° Centigrade (95° to 99° Fahrenheit) bearable; 25° to 30° Centigrade (77° to 86° Fahrenheit) pleasant; 15° Centigrade (59° Fahrenheit) cold; while 10° to 12° Centigrade (50° to 53° Fahrenheit) in a few minutes gives an extremely cold feeling.' To which he adds: 'For sedentary occupation he secures a temperature approximating to 33° Centigrade (91° Fahrenheit) around his skin by means of clothing and artificial heating; constantly trying to remove himself from the increase of cold which would increase heat production, his daily life is spent practically under the influence of a tropical climate; only about 20 per cent of his body is exposed to the air . . . Custom and fashion impose on the people clothing which is either unsuitable in character or too much. The great error is lack of ventilation. Too heavy clothing is less of an evil than badly ventilated clothing, because the latter provokes excessive sweating and leaves the skin needlessly long in active state. Clothing should allow great adaptability of body to change of temperature. It should not provoke sweating in the resting subject in still air at too low a temperature, e.g. at 27° Centigrade (80° Fahrenheit) instead of 30° Centigrade (86° Fahrenheit) . . . It is absurd that on a hot summer day boy scouts should march with a coloured scarf knotted round the neck, or invalid soldiers in Egypt wear a button-up shirt and a red tie. Nothing should be worn for ornament or smartness which increases the difficulty of losing heat and keeping down the body temperature. The avoidance of fatigue of the heart, the power to march, and the efficiency depend on prevention of heat stagnation.'

All of which was in line with the teaching of Sir Leonard's opposite number in Germany, Professor Max Rubner (1854–1932), the

Director of the Hygienic Institution in Berlin, whose *Handbuch der Hygiene*, which came out in six volumes between 1911 and 1913, was for long the standard book on the subject. According to Professor Rubner: 'Every hindrance to heat loss either reduces bodily exertion or causes the exertion to be done under a feeling of oppression and a burden of weariness.'

Before discussing the practical applications of this background information, a note on three of the most popular misconceptions in this field of clothing and climate may be interpolated: the topi; the spinal pad, and the cholera belt.

According to one of the most beloved and quoted of the Psalms (the 121st) of Holy Script, 'The sun shall not smite thee by day.' This concept of the danger of sunstroke, or *coup de soleil* as the French call it, dates back to very early times. The term itself is derived from the Latin *ictus solis*, based upon the Hippocratic teaching that certain cases of apoplexy were due to strokes of the sun. According to Aristotle, at least one of the purposes of the brain was to cool the blood; hence another very good reason for protecting the head from the sun. Plato, on the other hand, did not hold with this special susceptibility of the brain and that therefore the head required special protection from the sun, and it is of interest that, whilst the Roman soldiers wore a helmet, which, incidentally, had a felt or sponge lining which could be dampened to keep the head cool in hot weather, Julius Caesar is said often to have led his troops bareheaded.

By and large, however, both Greeks and Romans held firmly to the belief that a cool head and warm feet were two of the essentials of healthy living. A view as true today though for a long time it was ignored by our legislators. So many were the complaints at one time from Members of Parliament that a Ventilation Committee was set up which asked Sir Leonard Hill to investigate the matter for them. The gist of his report was: 'In the Chamber of the House of Commons the ventilating current is driven up through the floor in such a way as to cool the members' feet, while their heads are exposed to more stagnant air. Cold feet and stuffy

A Change of Air

heads result – just the wrong condition for legislation . . . I was allowed to make experimental alterations in the system of ventilation in one part of the chamber; closing up the floor inlets there, I introduced air at the Gallery level. Under these conditions

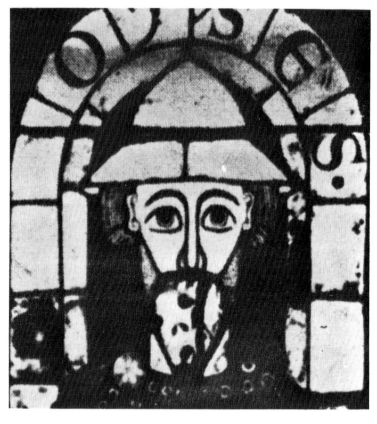

A solar topi depicted in the thirteenth-century stained glass windows of Augsburg Cathedral.

114

my feet were warm, my head agreeably cooled by a slight and grateful movement of the air.'

This belief in the necessity of protecting the head from the sun persisted all down the ages. It received confirmation from travellers to the East who reported that the natives 'wore great turbans to refract the sun beams.' What they failed to explain was why the womenfolk never wore them and yet were immune from sunstroke. The term, topi (the Hindu for hat), came into use last century as a result of the intense interest of the British army in protecting the troops from the sun. An infinite variety was introduced, one of the most widely used being the sola topi, so-called because it was made from pith; nothing to do with solar (from the sun). In *Wanderings of a Pilgrim in Search of The Picturesque*, published in 1850, Fanny Parkes describes one of the more exotic of these sola topis. 'The best sola hats are made in Calcutta; they are very light and form an excellent defence against the sun. At Meerut they cover them with the skin of pelicans with all the feathers on which renders it impervious to sun and rain, and the feathers sticking out beyond the brim of the hat give a demented view to the wearer.' In due course a neck curtain was added, which in time led to the spinal pad, which will be discussed shortly.

Eventually, as mentioned in chapter 7, the theory was evolved that it was the actinic rays of the sun, not the heat rays, that were responsible for what was then known as sunstroke, and we now call heatstroke as it is due to these heat rays. It was therefore logical, in the words of *The Lancet*, to line the topi with 'red to cut off these chemical or actinic rays to obviate the disastrous effects of the sun.' This was duly done, and received official approbation, though, it is interesting to note, Lord Roberts was not impressed with the suggestion. Not only were topis lined with red or orange, but orange underwear was also introduced for the troops, to protect them from 'the disastrous effects of the sun.' Again, official approbation was forthcoming until the United States Army got interested and carried out a carefully controlled trial in the

Philippines, the conclusion of which was that 'no beneficial effect whatever was observed from the use of this colour.'

The 1914–18 War more or less sounded the death-knell of the topi, though as late as 1920, Sir Leonard Hill was recommending for tropical wear 'a light sun helmet well ventilated and impermeable to sun rays.' The British in India, however, still clung to it as if it were part of the imperial heritage. In his fascinating reminiscences, *Unmade Journey*, published in 1977, Ian Stephen recalls how, when he first went to India in 1930: 'My father was very generous, indeed needlessly lavish in providing me with what was thought a proper outfit. I think he relished my "going East" because he'd himself done so when young . . . I remember particularly a white sun-helmet of strange shape in a japanned metal case, which I believe I never donned, and which embarrassed me for many years.' He recalls, however, the Viceroy, Lord Irwin, at a viceregal garden party 'raising his white "sola topi" in greeting his guests.' An even more interesting comment is that on an expedition in 1934 which took him to 12 000 feet. 'I had on me all that then in the early 1930s was thought proper for a European to wear on such an expedition. Pith-helmet or sola topi, of course, khaki-coloured. We all had to use them, anyway; there was supposedly a grave risk of sunstroke otherwise.'

They had not been completely obliterated, however, by the 1939–45 War and were used by the South African and Italian troops in the Abyssinian campaign, but soon gave way to the Australian slouch hat for those who wanted some protection from the heat of the sun. In *Charlie Company*, in which Peter Cochrane brilliantly describes his experiences as a 2nd lieutenant in the Queen's Own Cameron Highlanders in North Africa in 1940, he records: 'The Jocks wore nothing much but identity discs and a balmoral to keep the sun off; somewhere along the line topees or sun helmets had been slung away as lumber. I discarded mine as quickly and unobtrusively as possible, glad to be rid of the most awkward headgear ever devised by a military costumier. As children in the East my sister and I were smacked if we ventured

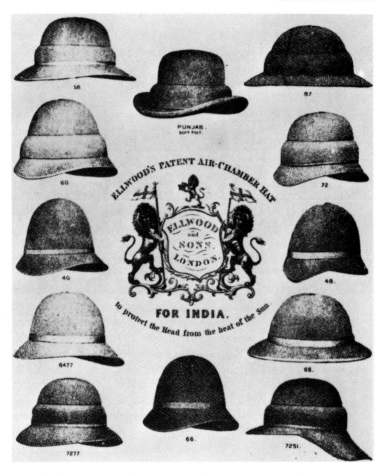

Various patterns of late nineteenth-century tropical headgear.

out without a topee, and it was heartening to find that the sun's lethal rays were a myth.' The one solitary proponent of the topi, who refused to give it up, was General Orde Wingate of the

117

Chindits: a characteristically exotic action on his part. According to the official *History of the Second World War*: 'There was difference of opinion as to the need of protective topis and spine pads. Some called them relics of superstition,' while the 1954 version of the official *Manual of Army Health* expressed the cautious view that 'it is now considered unlikely that the influence on body cooling afforded by headgear is sufficient to delay the onset of heatstroke, especially in the absence of other safety measures.'

The human race, however, is utterly unpredictable where fashions are concerned. While this book was being written a report in *The Times*, referring to a well-known firm of London tropical outfitter, stated: 'One unexpected feature of the firm's business: after almost disappearing for some years, topis are again in demand.' So that, like Panama hats and strawboaters, it looks as if they were going to surface again for the benefit of the manufacturers and the satisfaction of those who have more money than sense.

As has already been mentioned, in India the protection of the topi was often supplemented by a neck curtain to protect the back of the neck, and by the time of the Indian Mutiny the use of such a 'curtain' was fairly widespread. Gradually the concept spread that the spinal cord, as well as the brain, should be protected from the sun. So widespread did the belief become that Surgeon General Sir Joseph Fayrer, of the Indian Medical Department, when attached to the suite of Edward, Prince of Wales, during his tour of India in 1875, recorded that all the Prince's party were 'provided with light clothing and with quilted pads along the spine.'

It was not, however, until 1909 that they ('Pads, back, for European non-commissioned officers') were officially adopted by the British Army – in ample time to be included, along with the topi, in the commissariat supplies of our troops in Mesopotamia in the 1914–18 War. There, according to Sir William Willcox, consulting physician to the Mesopotamian Expeditionary Force, 'spinal pads 9 inches wide were necessary for the protection of the spinal cord from the sun's rays.' After the Mesopotamian fiasco

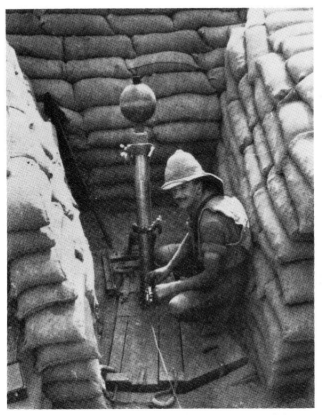

Soldier wearing a triangular spine pad and a neck curtain while preparing
a trench mortar in Mesopotamia during World War I.

little was heard of them, although they were still included in the
1936 *Official Regulations for the Clothing of The Army*, described as
'spine protectors', and were still being produced in Great Britain in
1940. To what extent they ever saw the light of day is unknown,
though there is some evidence that they occasionally surfaced in
India up to 1942.

Belts and girdles have a long and ancient history. Why the human race first started sporting them, and why they are as widespread today as they were in the heyday of Babylon and Egypt, is one of those mysteries of life which has aroused some of the more bizarre speculations on the part of psychologists and sociologists. According to Dr E. T. Renbourn, one factor was that from the earliest days 'travellers from Europe to the East were amazed at what the natives wore and assumed that it must have a hygienic purpose. The turban and its prolongation down the neck became the sun helmet and neck curtain and spine pad . . . The cummerbund [from the Persian, *Kamberband*, a loin cloth] of a number of tropical races was undoubtedly the forerunner of the flannel belt.'

Without doubt one reason, if not the main one, for the persistence of the flannel belt (or belly binder, to use its more homely connotation) was the well-recognised association between diarrhoea and feeling cold. Which was cause, and which was effect, was unknown, but what the ordinary human being soon realised was that the discomfort and chilly feeling of diarrhoea was relieved by the application of a nice tight warm belly binder – just as it often provided relief from the pain of colic. A point appreciated by that wise, if unqualified, physician, John Wesley, whose remedy for 'an habitual cholic' was: 'Wear a thin, soft flannel on the part.'

This association with diarrhoea was responsible for the popularity of the flannel binder when, in 1848, it was laid down that 'each soldier is to be provided with two cholera belts, as part of his necessaries.' The derivation of the new title is obvious: as often as not diarrhoea, or dysentery, in India meant cholera. And from now onwards the name stuck. For the next half-century the Army authorities in India swore by them, but gradually the onslaught of scientific medicine, in the form of the discovery of the specific microbic origin of diarrhoea (e.g., the *Vibrio cholerae* in the case of cholera) eroded faith in their value, and the last official reference to them appeared in Army regulations in 1911.

This, however, is by no means the end of the story. The cholera belt, or belly binder, may not be a cure for dysentery of specific bacterial origin, but it can still be a useful 'medical comfort', literally as well as metaphorically. And often, to comfort is still one of the prime purposes of the doctor – or at least ought to be. But let the experts speak for themselves.

In his justifiably popular textbook, *Clinical Physiology*, which ran into thirteen editions, in 1927 Professor R. J. S. McDowall, for many years Professor of Physiology at King's College, London, wrote: 'The wearing of so-called cholera belts signifies the importance of keeping this particular region of the body (the abdomen) warm, for the alimentary canal is a region especially liable to be infected as a result of cold. The production of diarrhoea or the return of symptoms after an attack of dysentery, which may follow a cold bath or sea-bathing, has long been recognised.' Some ten years later, *Hints to Travellers*, published by the Royal Geographical Society, commented: 'A drop in the night temperature in the tropics constitutes another danger, so protect the abdomen with warm clothing at night-time . . . Consider also the liability to chill and whether the often derided cholera belt is essential.' In 1952, a well-known textbook of tropical medicine stated that 'attacks of diarrhoea are often associated with chill of the abdomen especially at night when a light blanket or shawl should be wrapped round the abdomen and chest.'

Based on his experience during the 1939–45 War, a naval officer advised that on entering a hot climate suddenly or by air, the change from thick to thin clothes should be gradual, an undervest worn, and exercise avoided until acclimatisation was achieved. During residence a bush-shirt, or loose-fitting shirt with cellular underwear should be worn, with a change to thick clothes before sundown. An undervest should still be worn. Cool drinks should be sipped slowly. Finally, 'by night, a cholera belt or blanket folded across the abdomen should be worn with or without bedclothes.'

Writing in 1972, Dr Renbourn records that 'the abdominal belt is still issued to the Chelsea Pensioners who find it "comforting".'

And quite rightly. There are few things more comforting than a nice firm belly binder. It provides warmth and a sense of firmness that appeal to many – even in health. This is quite different from the unjustifiable permanent wearing of corsets to support the abdominal wall. In the healthy young, of either sex, no such support is required, and the practice should be discouraged. Even in the middle-aged, emphasis must always be laid on the importance of keeping the abdominal muscles firm and in good trim by exercise. But over and above this, there is still a real justification for the abdominal binder, whatever it may be made of and whatever its colour. It is not its constituent matter or its colour that matters. It is the support it gives, and the soothing warmth it imparts that make it such a valuable means to comfortable living.

All of which brings us to the present day and the problem of what we should wear in different climes. In the past, prior importance was given to the type of material clothes were made from. Wool, cotton, linen and silk all had their advocates. In due course big business came on the scene and, with the aid of the publicity wallahs, put forward the merits of their respective wares with that ingenuity whereby the skilled writer and designer of advertising copy can endow their clients' goods with the most fantastic properties without breaking the law.

What was overlooked was that the actual material was of little practical importance. Wool might feel warm, and linen might feel cool, whilst silk had the glamour and snob value bestowed by being expensive. All this, however, is secondary to two major factors: the texture of the material and its thickness. This point is best, and most conveniently, illustrated by two quotations from publications half a century apart.

In 1920, Sir Leonard Hill wrote: 'The claimants for systems all wool, linen, etc., have based their claims on the nature of the material – on the fibre – while the properties of a garment depend almost wholly not on the fibre, but on the manner of its weaving, and the same results can be secured with wool, cotton or linen by weaving out of each a material with the same porosity and air-holding power, permeability to moving air, and water-evaporating power . . . Wool next the skin is warmer because it is thicker than a smooth fine cotton or linen garment. A fine linen handkerchief lets ten times more heat through than a flannel shirt because of its thinness. Weave the linen equally thick and porous (air-holding) and it is as warm. Thin dry cotton flannelette is no less warm than flannel. The flannel is the warmer when wet, but the clothes of the citizen are rarely wet.'

In 1972, Dr E. T. Renbourn, in *Materials and Clothing in Health and Disease*, one of the most intriguing books written on the subject, whose scope is admirably described in its subtitle, 'History, Physiology and Hygiene. Medical and Psychological Aspects', wrote: 'Nowadays a struggle is still taking place between natural and synthetic fibres, it being claimed that because certain fibres are found in plants or animals, they are *natural* and therefore of necessity have virtues over those of synthetic fibres which, presumably, are *unnatural* . . . Under ordinary conditions there is not much to choose between the functional value of natural and synthetic fibres used as conventional fabrics . . . Not only can synthetic fibre material be blended with other fibres, but wool and cotton materials etc. are themselves often impure in nature. In fact, throughout history, cotton, wool, and linen have often been mixed with other fibres. Furthermore, with the large number of chemical and physical treatments to which most yarns and materials are exposed, the word *natural* no longer applies to so-called *natural* fibre fabrics. In fact, the word *biological* is much more applicable than the word *natural*. In the same way, synthetic fibres are sometimes treated by physical or chemical agents so that the properties of the resulting materials correspond somewhat to those of wool or cotton. In other words *synthetic* fibres may have some *natural* properties.'

The important factor, in other words, is not the material but the fabric. The real insulation of clothing is provided by the air entrapped within, or rather between and around, the fibres. This involves two considerations. One is that clothes should be loose, as has been the custom all down the ages until Victorian days in the case of the ladies, though somewhat earlier in the case of the menfolk. The Romans recognised the benefits of loose clothing with their togas, and the Arabs still do in hot climes, and the Eskimos in cold climes. The Church in this respect has set an excellent example, the traditional garb of monks and nuns illustrating the use of loose functional clothing.

The second means whereby this entrapment of air can be obtained is by means of so-called cellular clothing, particularly in the making of underwear. The extreme example of this was the string, or fish-net, underwear introduced by the Norwegian, Captain Brynje, and made of coarse string, loosely knitted with large holes in it. The enthusiasm with which these string vests were greeted has worn somewhat thin, and there is some evidence to justify the description of them as being too much of a good thing, or overdoing it. On the other hand, the general consensus of opinion is that 'cellular' underwear is best. Whether 'cellular' shirts offer additional advantage is problematical.

To pretend that there are complicated rules for clothing in different climes would be misleading, except in the case of those exposed to extremes of heat or cold, as in the tropics or in polar regions. In temperate climes, the minimum of clothing should be worn, consistent with feeling comfortable. This should be made of light-weight material. To adapt to changeable weather, extra garments should be worn, or discarded, according to weather conditions. A point to bear in mind in both hot and cold spells is that the air warmed by the skin rises by convection. Thus, in a hot spell immediate relief will be obtained by loosening the clothes round the neck – a common male practice in offices nowadays, though apparently frowned upon in New York. At least, according to a report from New York in *The Times* of 28 July 1977, 'an employee of IBM wrote a letter to his house journal suggesting that the corporation should review its "dress code" for June, July, August. "An open neck would be helpful. Why have we been stuck with jackets and ties while women wear casual and cool clothes?".' According to the report, written in the midst of the hottest July the United States had experienced since the dust bowl years of the 1930s, 'IBM thanked him for his suggestion but declined to adjust its attitude towards apparel. "To deviate significantly from normal business attire", the company replied, "does not seem appropriate".' Conversely, in cold weather this exitus of hot air round the neck should be closed by means of a muffler. Out of doors in cold windy weather the entrance of cold air round the wrists or the ankles should be reduced by wearing garments which seal off both wrists and ankles.

In cold climes the Eskimo sets the right example. His stock wear is a fur vest, drawers and socks with the hair towards the body, covered by a two-piece garment made of seal or caribou skin, consisting of a loose hooded jacket and long trousers. He wears mittens (not gloves) of the same material as his under-garments. The dress is the same for both sexes. With different material this should form the basis of all clothing for really cold climes. In view of modern air-conditioning the clothing must be flexible and adaptable, and the modern tendency on going out of doors is to don pullovers or quilted garments with an outer windproof layer made of the same synthetic material as is used for the quilting. Such a garment is warm and lightweight. This may be supplemented, or, in less cold conditions, replaced by the currently popular anorak. As already noted, all possible exists of warm air, and entrances for cold air, such as neck, wrists and ankles, must be firmly sealed.

'In principle,' it has been said, 'clothing for hot climates should consist of as few layers as possible, and made from very thin materials.' The old prejudice against nylon in hot climes dies hard, but there is no evidence that it is any less effective or comfortable than the cellular type of underwear. Underwear, however, should be worn. According to Dr Renbourn, 'a case has been made for the use of synthetic fibres or synthetic fibre blends for underclothing in the tropics. These should be worn with absorptive-fibre garments, e.g., a cotton shirt.' In his opinion, 'it is doubtful whether cellular cotton material is in any way cooler than thinner tight weave cotton, poplin, which helps to keep out biting insects.' The practical advantages of 'synthetic materials and blends (with fine wool, linen or cotton)' to which he draws attention are that 'they can be made very thin and have good wear qualities and excellent drip-dry and crease-resistant properties.'

All clothing should be loose, and the open neck should not be closed by a scarf or in any other way. If a suit is worn, this should be of light synthetic material and without any lining. Outer clothing should be of some light colour, white or yellow, to obtain maximum reflection of the sun's rays.

12

Climate and the heart

'Man may escape disease, but he cannot entirely escape climate. Normal man is able to adapt to the most rigorous environmental conditions; however, aged or diseased man does not tolerate hot and humid environments and may even be killed by climatic stress.' So wrote a well-known United States cardiologist, and of all the diseases particularly susceptible to climatic changes, those of the heart are the most important. Whether in health or ill health, the heart bears the ultimate strain and, as Professor W. E. Petersen, the outstanding proponent of climatology in the United States, put it once: 'Of all the factors and impacts to which the circulatory mechanism must adjust, for us, in a region of great meteorological variability, weather is for practical purposes the most important . . . As long as we must adjust to violent shifts in the air mass in which we exist, we will tax the vasomotor system to the limit and in so doing it will be inevitable that coronary dysfunction and coronary thrombosis [a heart attack in lay language] will occur.' All of which was put rather more simply and concisely by Hippocrates some two thousand years ago: 'The progress of the blood through the body proving irregular, all kinds of irregularities occur.'

It was also Hippocrates who warned his students that 'whoever has to pursue properly the science of medicine must proceed thus.

First he ought to consider what effects each season of the year can produce, for the seasons are not alike, but differ widely both in themselves and at their changes. For with the seasons men's diseases, like their digestive organs, suffer change.'

Which particular climatic factors affect the heart, and how, are still not quite clear. Extremes of heat and cold undoubtedly play a part, as does humidity. The effect of barometric pressure is not quite so clear, and there is a tendency to play it down, but a note published in the *British Medical Journal* some fifty years ago from an anonymous, but obviously observant, general practitioner is worthy of mention.

'About forty years ago,' he wrote, 'I began to notice that three elderly women with "heart trouble" used to send for me to visit them almost on the same day; they had no knowledge of each other. I next observed that their messages used to arrive when the barometer was unusually high. Ever since then I have been interested in similar observations. On November 19 [1925] a friend told me he had had word that morning of three deaths within his circle, two certainly from "heart failure". The same day I saw in *The Times* announcements of several sudden deaths "from heart failure", definitely so stated in two cases. The attention of the whole world has been riveted on the death of Queen Alexandra from "sudden heart attacks"; today *The Times* death column contains notices of five cases of sudden death, three of which are stated to be due to "heart failure". For the past week the barometer has stood remarkably high in England, particularly the South and East. I feel convinced that there is more than coincidence here, but I cannot advance any satisfactory explanation.'

Neither could the *British Medical Journal*, but in an annotation based on figures supplied by Dr Percy Stocks, then medical officer to the Department of Applied Statistics and Eugenics of London

University, it supported the anonymous reader's 'conviction that there was more than coincidence here.' Reviewing Dr Stocks' figures, which were based on data from Greenwich from 1900, it noted 'an appreciable relation between deaths from heart disease and atmospheric pressure', but drew attention to the proviso that 'since a high barometric pressure in November is often associated with a low temperature, which is known to increase mortality from heart disease, this might be the explanation.' On further statistical analysis, however, the conclusion was reached that 'there does appear to be a small but significant relation between heart deaths and atmospheric pressure during November apart from the effect of temperature.'

Since then, however, the emphasis has always tended to be on the adverse effects of heat and cold. Thus, Professor Petersen concluded that 'coronary thrombosis is characteristically seasonal, occurring most often during periods of unusually high or low temperature, and most often after periods of cold.' To illustrate his point he quotes the deaths of two United States Presidents: Calvin Coolidge and Franklin D. Roosevelt. The former died suddenly of a coronary thrombosis on 5 January 1933. His death was preceded by a severe cold wave that reduced the temperature to 60° F. (15.5° C.) on one day. The temperature then rose as abruptly as it had fallen and, according to Professor Petersen, it was this combination that caused the fatal presidential heart attack.

President Roosevelt's death was somewhat more complicated. On 25 March 1945, he had a very severe 'cerebral episode' at his home at Hyde Park, N.Y. He was rushed to Warm Springs, Georgia, where he died on 12 April. At Hyde Park the temperature had reached the 80°s F. (around the late 20°s C.) in mid-March and then fell sharply to freezing levels by 22 March. Then came an upswing with an occluded front (i.e. temperature up and barometric pressure also increasing). 'Under these weather conditions,' according to Professor Petersen, 'Mr Roosevelt experienced a serious cerebral accident, a "stroke".' At Warm Springs there was a related situation. It was almost freezing on 7

April; 'then an uprising of 40° F. (22° C.) and, with this, the terminal episode.'

This correlation of strokes with external temperature is well recognised, though not so well documented. It is an association that one expects as, in the words of Hippocrates, a stroke is but another example of the 'progress of the blood through the body proving irregular', which he elaborates by saying: 'So in one place it [the blood] stops, in another it passes sluggishly, in another more quickly.' Two relatively recent reports, one from Belfast and one from Yugoslavia, confirm the association, the Belfast evidence, based on 1016 cases of stroke, indicating that the correlation was most marked over the age of fifty. The Yugoslavian report, which is more detailed meteorologically, and based on a series of 463 strokes seen between 1950 and 1960, has this as one of its conclusions. 'The greatest number of strokes (65 per cent) appear during the development of a southern "front" without pre-cipitation [rainfall] or a northern "front" with precipitation. A smaller number are seen during the development of a southern "front" with precipitation, and the least number during the development of a northern "front" without precipitation.' This conclusion is quoted in full as it indicates the complexity that still surrounds any attempt to solve the riddle of the association of climate and disease, and indicates the need for a much more intensive onslaught from doctors, meteorologists, physicists and astronomers alike.

Of the association between cold and coronary artery disease, however, there is no doubt. How precisely cold affects the coronary arteries and drives them into spasm is not quite clear. The effect is associated with the constriction of the blood-vessels of the skin induced by cold, as already discussed in chapter 6. Two obvious possibilities are that either this constriction of the skin blood-vessels induces a rise in blood pressure which puts an extra strain on a faulty coronary system, or skin and coronary artery constriction (or spasm) occur together. Whatever the mechanism, the result is definite and precise. In the earlier stages of coronary disease, this spasm induces the intense pain under the sternum (or chest bone) known as angina pectoris. This pain, which often radiates down the left arm, is the consequence of the myocardium, as the heart muscle is known, being deprived of oxygen as a result of an inadequate blood supply, and going into spasm. The most common precipitant of this agonizing pain is exercise, and it is characteristic of this dreaded pain that it gradually goes when the afflicted individual rests. In other words it is a warning from Nature that the heart is being asked to do more than it is capable of and that, unless the strain is taken off the heart, it will crack up.

Sudden cold may also bring on the pain – and for the same reason: spasm of the coronary arteries with a consequent insufficient blood supply to the heart muscle. In some people, opening the door on first going out in the morning may bring on an attack, as may opening the door of the kitchen refrigerator. This is why the individual (usually a male) subject to angina pectoris must always keep himself warm, both in and out of doors. Thus, his bedroom must be comfortably warm before he goes up to it at night and before he gets up in the morning. Similarly his bed must always be warm – to him an electric blanket is a necessity, not a luxury. Equally, he must wear ample warm clothing before he ventures out in cold weather, and must realise that a low temperature, particularly with a cold wind, will reduce his exercise tolerance very considerably.

As the coronary arteries become increasingly inefficient the possibility of a heart attack becomes more likely, though many patients continue to live quite happily for long periods provided they keep their daily requirements within the limitations imposed by the heart: in other words, the heart rules the roost, not vice versa. The precise mechanism of these heart attacks, which can occur without any previous angina pectoris, is not quite clear, but for all practical purposes it boils down to an important branch of the coronary arteries becoming permanently blocked: hence the term, coronary thrombosis. (Incidentally the coronary arteries owe their name to the fact that, before plunging down into the substance of the heart muscle, they circle round the base of the heart in the form of a crown.) While this closure, which, it should be noted, is only fatal in a minority of cases, may be associated with exercise, including exercise in the cold, such as shovelling snow; it may also occur while the victim is resting – either in a chair or in bed. But, whenever and however it occurs, it is more likely to do so in the cold season, and therefore correspondingly more caution must be exercised during the winter.

Even so, however, the problem still exists of what precise climatic changes induce these heart attacks. Typical of the problem involved is a report from Dallas, Texas, with its 'quite hot summers, rather mild winters and the frequent occurrence of sudden changes in temperature and humidity.' An analysis was made of the relationship between these sudden changes in weather and the 1386 cases of heart attacks due to coronary artery disease admitted to three Dallas hospitals during a five-year period. This revealed an increased frequency of such cases during periods of sudden inflow of polar or of tropical air masses. In discussing these findings the authors of the report comment that the exact mechanism by which sudden changes of weather may be related to the occurrence of what they technically describe as acute myocardial infarction is unknown.

'Rapid onset of either hot or cold weather is always accompanied by simultaneous changes in wind velocity and direction as well as barometric pressure changes . . . Cold is not the only meteorological factor which may be important. Many of the patients had the onset of their symptoms either indoors, in a warm environment, during sleep or at rest. About half of the cases occurred during the early period of polar inflow, when the temperature was still falling and the barometric pressure was continuing to rise. The facts suggest that other meteorological factors, possibly including changes in barometric pressure, are operating in addition to decreased temperature alone. The increase in barometric pressure during polar inflows averaged 0.53 inch or 13.97 millimetres of mercury. It is possible that abrupt changes in barometric pressure of this magnitude may exert an important influence in the precipitation of acute myocardial infarction.'

Some twenty years later, a comparable opinion was expressed in a report from Israel. 'Our findings confirm the association of short-term fluctuations in cardiac mortality with weather changes. Specifically, low temperature and high barometric pressure appear to be of primary significance; low wind velocity and, to a lesser extent, relative humidity appear to be additive to the former. Taken together, the results of the analysis thus far completed suggest that the transitional period of turbulent atmospheric conditions preceding an intrusion of a cold wave and the following stabilisation of anticyclonic weather with below normal temperature, elevated barometric pressure and low wind velocity constitute a sequence of events at which increases in cardiac mortality are most often noted'.

The effect of high temperatures on the heart have already been discussed in chapter 7. The strain of a hot humid atmosphere on the heart, particularly on the damaged heart, has been particularly studied by Professor G. E. Burch in New Orleans, whose climate is characterised by mild winters and hot humid summers. Typical of the New Orleans figures are those for 1952–55, when, of the 1582 cases of coronary thrombosis admitted to the Charity Hospital, the highest monthly incidence was in August, and the lowest in December, whereas in northern U.S. cities, such as Philadelphia, New York and Cincinnati, the highest incidence was in January and February. The reason why the incidence is not higher in the summer in northern cities such as New York, which can produce quite unpleasant heat waves, is probably that these heat waves are of comparatively short duration and that during the summer the relatively cool nights relieve the heart of the burden of heat stress, whereas in New Orleans there tends to be no, or relatively little, let-up at night. Another possible explanation is that patients with heart trouble become acclimatised to the hot humid conditions. There is certainly evidence that the death rate from heart attacks is lower in the second and subsequent heat waves than in the first one, particularly if the latter is of sudden onset and occurs fairly early in the summer.

The effect of a hot humid environment was dramatically illustrated by Professor Burch in an experiment with human guinea-pigs that he was brave enough to carry out. He submitted twelve hospital patients with mild heart failure and thirteen patients with normal hearts to a temperature of 104° F. (40° C.) and a relative humidity of 85 per cent in a climatic laboratory. When the patients were first put in the laboratory the temperature was 73° F. (23° C.) and the relative humidity was 60 per cent. These were quickly raised to the experimental level in a quarter of an hour. In other words no time was allowed for acclimatisation to the hot humid environment. In ten of the twelve patients with heart failure the heart was so badly affected by the experimental hot humid conditions that, in Professor Burch's own words, this 'necessitated immediate return to comfortable conditions to avoid serious consequences. In five of them the failure was extreme.' Fortunately, he notes, 'in most instances all subjects returned to their respective previous basal states within an hour or two.'

Some sixteen years later he attempted to repeat the experiment in a modified manner, exposing comparable patients to a temperature of 90° F. (32° C.) and a relative humidity of 75 per cent but the attempt to expose them to these conditions had to be given up because they were too stressful. The experiment was then carried out at the same temperature but a relative humidity of only 41 per cent: in other words, a hot dry clime. The mean duration during which patients with and without heart failure were exposed to these conditions was 6·8 days (ranging from four to twelve days). The interesting, practical finding was that 'in general the patients with heart failure were more uncomfortable' than those with healthy hearts and they did not become acclimatised to the hot dry conditions as did the healthy patients. From which the practical conclusion is drawn that 'patients with heart failure living in tropical or subtropical climates cannot depend on full acclimatisation to cope satisfactorily with heat stress. These patients should be advised to reduce their physical activities in order to decrease the rate of heat production and to live in a cool, comfortable or air-conditioned environment to facilitate heat loss.'

The value and importance of air-conditioning are admirably exemplified in a study of deaths during heat waves in St Louis. One hospital was divided into three main units, only one of which was air-conditioned. Each patient was confined to one of the three units. All thirty-five deaths due to heart failure caused by the heat wave occurred in the two units without air-conditioning.

In a monograph on *Cardiovascular Disease in The Tropics*, published by the British Medical Association, Professor Burch amplifies his advice. Patients with mild heart disease are advised to spend several days relatively free from physical exercise following initial exposure to a hot humid environment. Meals should be small and frequent with a liberal intake of fluids and ample salt. Clothing should be light and loose and 'air movement should be assured.' Whenever possible, air-conditioning adjusted for the comfort of the individual should be employed. When physical activity is resumed this must be done cautiously with frequent periods of rest. 'This same advice,' it is pointed out, 'is also beneficial to healthy people.' Those with more serious types of heart disease 'must exercise extreme caution in hot, humid conditions.' Even washing dishes in hot water or simply being in a room where clothes are being laundered 'may constitute an intolerable stress for such patients.' Such patients, as already noted, acclimatise badly. Air-conditioning is said to be 'most effective' – some would say essential – for their proper management.

In contrast to Professor Burch's sophisticated human experiments in the United States of America, and even more striking as evidence of the harmful effect of a hot humid environment, is the natural human experiment carried out in Nigeria. Here, as elsewhere, the number of patients with heart failure admitted to hospital is much higher in the hot wet months, when the temperature may reach 104° F. (40° C.) and the relative humidity rises to around 70 per cent, but there is an interesting complicating factor. This is the high incidence of heart failure following pregnancy in the womenfolk of two of the tribes. In these tribes the practice is that immediately after delivery, and for 40 to 120 days, the mother takes two scalding hot baths daily to keep out the 'cold', using a bundle of leaves to splash around 5 pints (30 litres) of very hot water over her body. Temperatures of 180° F. (82° C.) have been recorded immediately before the bathing process started. Not surprisingly, superficial burns are common. After this gruelling (or perhaps, grilling would be a more appropriate adjective) the unfortunate mother remains in a well-heated room, with a fire or glowing embers underneath a specially constructed dried mud bed which retains the heat for several hours.

A more effective way of inducing heat stress, and putting additional strain on the heart, could scarcely be imagined, and it is anything but surprising that so many of these mothers become dropsical as a result of a failing heart. And all this rigmarole is carried out in 'an attempt to prevent cold (*sanyi*) from entering the body' as cold is thought to be a common cause of illness, and especially puerperal diseases, including dropsy. It is interesting that similar ideas about cold prevail in Malaysia.

To come back from these primeval beliefs and practices to the more humdrum life of western civilisation, the hazards of heat, even in this much vaunted scientific age, are exemplified in a recent report from the United States, based primarily on a study of the state of affairs in the summers of 1946–75. This shows that during one day in July in the heat wave of 1966, the death rate in the 'urban core' of St Louis was $5\frac{1}{2}$ times greater than in the nearby suburbs. On the same day, 1020 deaths were recorded in the New York, New Jersey metropolitan area, an excess of 539 over the expected number for that day, while the two-week heat wave of this year 'took the lives of approximately 1181 citizens of New York City who would have normally lived beyond the summer of

1966.' The aged, the poor, and diabetics, as well as those with heart and lung disease, had considerably higher mortality rates than the general population.

This reference to the aged is important. Whatever the state of their hearts, they are much more susceptible to heat, as to cold, than the younger members of the population, and all too often a heat wave reveals the first evidence of a failing old heart. The ageing heart may be able to cope with the ordinary demands of an equable climate, but the moment an extra strain is put on it, as by a hot humid environment, it begins to falter. Hence the importance of ensuring that the elderly are living in conditions in which extremes of heat (and cold) can be controlled.

Before concluding this chapter, brief reference may be made to some recent interesting developments in our knowledge as to how climate affects the heart. The most recent, and interesting, is the suggestion that one method whereby a hot clime may affect the heart is by inducing an increased output of a hormone known as aldosterone. This is a hormone which plays an important part in fluid control in the body. According to recent reports, heating can directly stimulate production of aldosterone to 'an inordinately high level', and thereby induce retention of the sodium ion, which in turn puts an extra strain on the heart. In addition, high environmental temperatures stimulate the production of another hormone which cuts down the passage of urine, thereby putting yet another strain on the heart. It is also said to stimulate the thirst centres in the brain which control the desire to drink. Taken altogether, these three factors must obviously play a considerable part in inducing heart failure in hot humid conditions.

Of more academic interest, but demonstrating how the tangled skein of climate and health is being untangled, is the report from Romania that in mice an increase in air temperature and a lowering of barometric pressure cause a decrease in the amount of potassium ion in the heart muscle. This fits in with a previous report that at high altitude the record of the electrical activity of the heart, known as the electrocardiogram, is typical of that induced by a low level of potassium in the blood. The practical importance of this observation is that, as I was one of the first to show some forty years ago, the potassium ion plays an important role in the activity of the heart muscle, and either an excess or a lack of it, can have an adverse effect.

Finally there is the report from Hungary that the level of cholesterol in the blood of patients with arteriosclerosis (thickening of the arteries) was 'greatly influenced by meteorological factors.' A comparable report from Baltimore showed what was described as a 'highly significant seasonal variation in the blood cholesterol level' in twenty-four healthy young men: highest in the late spring, summer and early autumn. In view of what has been described as the 'current epidemic' of western civilisation of deaths due to ischaemic heart disease, which results from disease of the arterial wall, and the correlation of this with cholesterol, these are observations which clearly demand further investigation.

As a postscript, a brief reference may be made to mounting evidence that there is a correlation between the weather and the clotting of blood. The tendency to clotting seems to be increased with the passage of warm and cold fronts. According to one Danish observer, 'the velocity of the changes in barometric pressure seems to be the only really important factor, i.e. the faster the changes in barometric pressure, the greater the biological effect.' Be that as it may, this is yet another facet of the subject of this book that has never been fully investigated. Of its importance there can be no doubt because, whilst a clot in the leg may be of little more than nuisance value (though quite unpleasant), a clot circulating round the body may prove lethal if it lands in some vital point such as the lungs, heart, or brain. To the surgeon the possibility of a fatal pulmonary embolism, as a clot in the lung is technically known, is a perpetual nightmare. Many of these cases have hitherto been considered inexplicable. Might it be that this is because no-one has thought of studying the possible association with climatic changes?

Where should patients in this country with heart disease seek relief and obtain the best possible climatic conditions in which to derive the maximal enjoyment of life within their cardiac limitations? The answer, which can scarcely be improved upon, was given by a well-known London heart specialist some forty years ago. 'They should be advised to winter, if possible, in a warm climate at a moderate altitude, or, preferably, at sea level. Suitable places in England include Bournemouth, Torquay, Sidmouth, Paignton, etc. on the south coast, or, if the patient prefers and can afford it, he may winter abroad in Madeira, the Canary Islands, Egypt or Algiers.' To which might be added South Africa and the West Indies.

13

Climate and asthma and bronchitis

The association between climate and asthma is played down in Britain in this era of so-called scientific medicine. This is partly because it is a somewhat ill-defined condition, partly because there is practically always a pyschological element in its causation, and to the modern laboratory-orientated doctor, which our medical schools are producing in ever-increasing numbers, such an element is frowned upon as it precludes his being able to prescribe a specific medicine which will produce a specific effect. To this generation of doctors climate comes into the same category as emotion as a vague, ill-defined entity incapable of classification into watertight compartments.

Typical of this approach is the fact that one of the most popular (and rightly so) textbooks of treatment for students never even mentions climate as a factor to be taken into consideration in dealing with asthma. Another equally popular textbook's only reference to the subject is to include 'acrid fumes and cold' among the 'non-specific factors' that may 'aggravate the symptoms.' A well-spoken-of textbook of children's diseases admits that 'in some cases climate and physical environment are so important in precipitating attacks that change of residence is justifiable', adding, however, with true Scottish caution, that 'every case must be investigated before such a change is advised.' The justification advanced in support of this note of caution is worth quoting in full. 'A full psychological history should be taken as well as an investigation of possible allergens [substances to which the individual is allergic and which produce an attack] in the home before it is assumed that a change of climate (e.g. from country to town in a pollen-sensitive patient, from mountains to sea or vice versa) will be beneficial. The number of cases in which change of climate is really necessary is quite small.'

How true is this last statement I know not, but the cautious approach is advisable in view of the multiplicity of factors involved in the causation of asthma. To go to all the expense of moving house and finding that there is no amelioration of the asthmatic attacks in the new surroundings is an experience from which the victims of the disease should be protected so far as is humanly possible. To experiment with ringing the climatic changes for short holiday spells is another matter, and it is in not encouraging such 'experiments' that British doctors do a disservice to their asthmatic patients.

The current standard British textbook of paediatrics sums up the position as follows. 'Weather factors which may influence the development of asthma include temperature, humidity, barometric pressure, wind velocity and air pollution.' No indication is given as to how often these factors come into play, but it is stated that 'in Britain climatic factors are undoubtedly important in precipitating asthmatic attacks in childhood, but it is seldom an easy matter to isolate the responsible factor, and there may be several.' In support of this last statement it refers to Dutch reports purporting to show a statistically significant relationship between the onset of asthmatic attacks and a sudden increase in general atmospheric turbulence, combined with the influence of cold air-masses. This, it adds, 'may be, and probably is, a simple physical matter – the sudden inhalation of cold air reflexly stimulating bronchospasm in susceptible individuals – but it has been suggested that such air movements could be the means whereby fungal spores from distant areas are brought into the patient's environment, there to act as allergens. Such a movement of fungal spores has been investigated and is well documented but the relationship of such spores to childhood asthma is less certain, and is probably of no very great importance.'

The Dutch finding of a correlation between asthmatic attacks and exposure to cold has been confirmed by subsequent research in the Netherlands, including a study of seventy-five children carried out over a year, which revealed that in winter and early spring the number of asthmatic attacks increased during periods of cooling. Similar observations have been made in Germany and the U.S.A., and the suggestion has been advanced that this sensitivity of asthmatics to changes in environmental cooling may be due to a poorly functioning thermoregulation mechanism. This is a suggestion that is supported by the finding that if the hand of an asthmatic is cooled, it takes longer to return to normal temperature than does the hand of a healthy individual.

That the problem, however, is not as simple as this is suggested by a report from Brisbane based on a study of the annual incidence there of asthma attacks over a seven-year period. According to this, 'the element most closely associated with asthma was rainfall. There was a minor, independent association with temperature and also with soil moisture. This combination is taken to support the hypothesis that the increase in asthmatic attacks in these circumstances is due to the production of allergens produced by the action of micro-organisms on decaying grass or other vegetation.' Be that as it may, these Brisbane findings fit in with a century-old British report that low damp areas with abundant vegetable life were unsuited for asthmatics.

A further complication brought out by this Brisbane report is the difficulty in deciding whether an improvement in the asthmatic state in response to a change of weather is directly due to the change or indirectly by virtue of the climatic change diminishing the number of allergens to which the individual is susceptible. The obvious example of this is the seasonal incidence, as in the case of hay fever, where it is not the weather that induces the symptoms, but the absence or presence of certain allergens. The weather plays only an indirect part by increasing, or decreasing, the amount of pollen to which susceptible individuals are exposed. Hence the value of the pollen count, a method that was introduced in the U.S.A. over fifty years ago to warn hay-fever subjects of the risk they ran of having an attack on any given day. Here the role of the weather is in deciding the local intensity of pollen, which is affected by climatic factors such as wind, humidity and the like. Incidentally, it is interesting to note that as long ago as 1873 a British doctor, who was himself a victim of hay fever, was recommending seaside resorts on the windward side of the country to his hay-fever patients as means of avoiding the dangerous pollen season.

Until these problems have been solved – and further work is urgently required on the subject, what is clear, judging from European experience, is that asthmatics are free from attacks in mountains at heights of around 5000 feet (1500 metres). At these altitudes, it has been said, the patient benefits not only from the climatic stress and adaptation but also from the purity of the air, which allows optimal conditions for the relief of catarrh and asthma. In altitudes of over 1500 metres the air is virtually free of allergens. At 5500 feet (1700 metres) elevation asthma is less bothersome. The low oxygen content of the air in high places causes a deepening and acceleration of breathing. These benefits were concisely summed up in one characteristically short sentence by Sir Leonard Hill: 'Alpine climate is almost a specific for asthma in children, the asthma clearing so long as they remain in this climate.'

This beneficial action of high altitudes in asthma is confirmed by the report of the Indian Army medical service already referred to, but they are more non-committal as to the prime factor responsible for the reduction in asthmatic attacks at the much higher altitudes (12 000 to 18 000 feet (3700 to 5500 metres)). Thus they include among the possible responsible factors: reduced partial pressure of oxygen, marked differences in summer and winter temperatures, low humidity, differences in the quality and intensity of solar radiation, differences in the ozone content of the air, and changes in the number of air ions.

This last factor is of particular interest in view of a report from Jerusalem of the apparently beneficial effect of negative air ions in asthmatic children. The experimental basis upon which this investigation was carried out was that 'under the influence of positive ions, a sensitive organism may develop a condition similar to that of an asthmatic attack.' As negative ions have an action antagonistic to that of positive ions, it was decided to study the effect of negative ions on thirteen children who had what is described as 'asthmatic bronchitis', and it is claimed that the negative air ions shortened the asthmatic attacks. To what extent this use of air ions has been carried into practice I have been unable to determine, but it is obviously a method deserving of careful consideration. It is at least safe, which is more than can be said of some of the anti-asthmatic drugs now being used. Further, there is evidence that air-ion treatment is of help in the management of hay fever, the other major allergic affliction of mankind.

Asthmatics are also being treated in low-pressure chambers at simulated altitudes of 6500 to 8200 feet (2000 to 2500 metres). Rapid improvement is claimed, and even 'cure', after a series of 60 to 100 treatments, particularly in younger asthmatics. This is a more rational adaptation of 'high-altitude' therapy than the one time vogue of taking asthmatics up in aeroplanes to heights of around 5000 feet to give them relief, a method, incidentally, which was even used at one time for the relief of the spasmodic attacks of whooping-cough.

In Germany much work has been done on treating asthmatic children at the seaside, where it is claimed that under the influence of clean, moist air, rich in salt, 'asthmatic difficulties are quickly resolved.' Although one German report claimed 'permanent relief' in 39 per cent of patients treated on the North Sea coast, the general consensus of opinion is that the improvement is temporary, just as it is in mountain therapy. That, however, is no fundamental criticism of the method. If asthmatics, particularly children, can obtain even temporary relief, combined with the other benefits of living a healthy open-air life under such conditions, then they will benefit in the long run. How much of the benefit is due to freedom from contact with offending allergens is difficult to assess. At both the coast and in the mountains allergens, as well as atmospheric pollutants, which are also liable to induce asthmatic attacks, are absent or negligible in number, and this is undoubtedly at least part of the explanation of the benefit asthmatics derive from holidays at the sea or in the mountains.

To come down to a more practical level for those asthmatics who are contemplating either a permanent change of residence in their search for relief, or a suitable holiday resort in this country, the advice given by Dr Edgar Hawkins in *Medical Climatology of England and Wales* in 1923 can scarcely be bettered. 'Asthma is a complaint for which it is always difficult to prescribe a climate with confidence. A mere change of residence from town to country, or from country to town, may give a temporary relief.' What is to be aimed at is 'fresh, dry air' and 'a good elevation'. Among his specific recommendations are the Channel Islands, Malvern, Grange-over-Sands, Bournemouth, the Isle of Wight, Sidmouth and Torquay. For undisclosed reasons he issues a warning against, amongst other places, Aberystwyth, the Lake District, and Rhyl (but not Colwyn Bay or Llandudno).

> 'Chronic bronchitis is the name given to the clinical syndrome which many individuals develop in response to the long-continued action of various types of irritant on the bronchial mucosa [lining membrane]. The most important of these is tobacco smoke, but they also include dust, smoke and fumes . . . Exposure to dampness, to sudden changes in temperature and to fog may be responsible for exacerbations of chronic bronchitis.'

> 'The fact that chronic bronchitis is more prevalent in Britain than in any other country in the world is mainly the result of

failure to control atmospheric pollution. Britain's generally damp and cold climate may, however, be an aggravating factor. The high humidity of the atmosphere not only reduces the rate of smoke dispersal but, by dissolving some of the irritant gases, such as sulphur dioxide and sulphur trioxide and converting them into acids, potentiates their action on the bronchial mucosa.'

These quotations from two currently popular textbooks summarise the current views on what has for long been known as the 'English disease' because of its higher incidence in this island home of ours than elsewhere. Why we should have this unpleasant record no-one knows. The suggestion that it is associated with our high degree of atmospheric pollution is no longer tenable. Neither can it be attributed to our smoking habits. As a nation we undoubtedly smoke more cigarettes than are good for us, but we are not so exceptional in this respect. Constitutional factors, which undoubtedly play a part and explain why some of us do not go down with the disease, are not likely to explain the national incidence. All of which suggests that our climate may be a dominating factor, but how dominating is anyone's guess.

What does seem to be clear from all the many investigations that have been carried out into the problem over the last century is that two important causative factors are cold and atmospheric pollution, the emphasis always tending to be placed on the former.

Thus, writing in 1924, on the basis of a review of London records dating back to 1870, W. T. Russell, the Chief Statistical Clerk of the National Institute for Medical Research, concluded that fog itself had no appreciable effect on the respiratory death rate but, 'whenever the prevalence of fog was associated with a depression in the temperature, then there was a rapid increase in the number of adult deaths.' In 1968, a report from St Thomas's Hospital confirmed the ill-effects of low temperature and atmospheric pollution noted by others, adding: 'The associations we have found give no indication of the mechanisms by which cold and atmospheric pollution produce their effects.'

In between, in more sense than one, came a report published in 1960, comparing the relationship between mortality from respiratory disease on the one hand and atmospheric pollution and meteorological conditions on the other in 1947–54 in East Anglia and London Administrative County. In both these areas a close correlation was found between a low temperature and a raised absolute humidity and death from lung and heart diseases in those aged forty-five years and over. Of the East Anglian findings the report says: 'It appears that the urban atmospheric pollution absent in East Anglia has little effect on the general association between temperature, humidity and mortality.' Of the effect of fog it says: 'It appears that the more serious effects of metropolitan fog, as measured by excessive increases in mortality occur only when fog is accompanied by very low temperature conditions.'

Although we are still fundamentally ignorant of why some people develop chronic bronchitis whilst others escape its grip, it does seem to be clear that, once having developed, the avoidance of cold damp climes and of atmospheric pollution is a wise step. As one current textbook puts it: 'Since atmospheric pollution is an undisputed cause of chronic bronchitis and some of its acute exacerbations, it would be logical to advise patients with this condition to move permanently to a region where pollution is absent or negligible and the climate warm and dry.' 'Unfortunately,' it adds, 'such favourable environment does not exist in any part of the United Kingdom and patients seeking it must go to the Mediterranean, South Africa, New Zealand or the West Indies. Such advice is very seldom economically or socially acceptable, but occasionally a move from a heavily polluted city to a country district may be practicable and, to a limited extent, beneficial.'

This is a reasonably judicial summing up of the situation, with one proviso. As already noted in chapter 3, the winter climate of the Mediterranean is not as reliable as some would make it out to be. To winter there may be worth considering, but to take up permanent residence is another matter. Many would also include the Canary Islands in the list – again for a winter holiday, though not necessarily for a permanent move.

So far as Britain is concerned, the most acceptable parts for the chronic bronchitic to settle are the Cornish coast around Falmouth, South Devon, Bournemouth, Eastbourne and the Channel Islands. The merits of some of these places are admirably summed up in the report of the Royal Medical and Chirurgical Society published in 1895, and referred to in chapter 1. Thus, of Bournemouth it says:

> 'The effect of the climate on the subjects of chronic bronchitis sent to Bournemouth for treatment is, in the opinion of most of the local observers, decidedly favourable. It is represented that winter cough in persons over fifty is kept in abeyance by residence here; that visitors with chronic bronchitis quickly improve and that the dry soil, the shelter afforded by a carefully selected residence, the sedative influence of the atmosphere, and the exhalation from the pines all contribute these effects.'

Of Devon it says:

> 'With regard to chronic bronchitis . . . persons who have been accustomed to spend the whole winter indoors and in whom the usual "winter cough" has lasted hitherto for months, on taking up their residence in Devonshire, find that they can spend the greater part of the day out of doors and that the duration of their attacks is reckoned by weeks instead of months.'

The over-all position is succinctly summed up by Dr Hawkins as:

> 'The choice must fall on a dry and equable spot (particularly in winter), without dust, and where regular exercise can be taken. If there is much secretion it is well to aim at a dry atmosphere, but with a harsh and irritable cough, a moister climate is more desirable.'

One further point is worth noting, as indicating that in many ways chronic bronchitis is the condition in which most benefit can be obtained from taking climatic factors into consideration. According to the textbook that has just been quoted, 'all patients who can do so should remain at home with the doors and windows closed during periods of fog. There is indeed much to be said for advising severe chronic bronchitics who are retired or unemployed to remain indoors throughout the winter.' This theoretically sound advice holds out a pretty bleak prospect for the unfortunate victim of bronchitis. Granted that the further comment is made that 'those who can afford to spend the winter abroad in a warm dry climate may derive great benefit from doing so', but such people are few and far between in these days of the much vaunted Welfare State, and are becoming rarer. What is obviously indicated therefore is that those with chronic bronchitis should give serious consideration to moving to a more salubrious part of the country where the chance of the civilian equivalent of 'C.B.' (Confined to Barracks) for the winter can be avoided. The cold night air may be bad for the chronic bronchitic, but God's fresh, mild, equable air is what he needs to get the optimum ease of breathing to which he aspires – and is entitled. And the move should not be left to too late a stage when the lungs are so badly damaged that relief is increasingly difficult to obtain. It should be made as soon as it is clear that the condition is present. At this stage change of climate will not cure, but the chances are that it will slow up, if not arrest, the progress of the disease process.

14

Climate and infection

'It seems likely that close investigation of the influence of climate and other environmental factors on the cause of epidemics might suggest practical measures of individual protection.' So wrote Sir Macfarlane Burnet, the distinguished Australian virologist, in 1940. Alas, medical scientists became so bemused with antibiotics and the intricacies of the defence mechanism of the body against disease that they had little or no time to devote to such old fashioned factors as climate. Yet the association between climate and infections has intrigued mankind, including its doctors, for century after century. Practically two hundred years ago, William Heberden, described by Samuel Johnson as 'the last of our learned physicians', published a notable article entitled 'Influence of Cold upon Health', based on shrewd personal observations of the patients entrusted to his care. It was by no means a new concept, but it presented the case for such an association in a clear, concise manner which set an example as to how such clinical evidence should be collected and presented.

A century later, certainly so far as infections were concerned, his teaching had been overwhelmed by the torrent of reports which followed Louis Pasteur's classical reports on the bacterial cause of disease. Tuberculosis, diphtheria, anthrax, cholera, and a host of other infectious diseases were shown to be due to specific micro-organisms. In their characteristic sheep-like manner the medical profession jumped on this bandwaggon, assuming that all that was now necessary was to find means of destroying these bacteria and all would be well. Undoubtedly much progress was achieved by the production of antitoxins and the like that killed some of these micro-organisms such as those of tetanus and diphtheria, but there were many others, against which we had no defence, except that provided by Nature, until the sulpha drugs and antibiotics were discovered some forty to fifty years on. In the interregnum the position was admirably summed up by the dictum concerning pneumonia current when I was a medical student. Seventy per cent of cases recover no matter what you do. Twenty per cent die no matter what you do. The remaining ten per cent you can do something to help – and that mainly by good nursing. And it might have been added that 'good nursing' involved nursing the patient by an open window; a half-hearted admission that climate, in the form of fresh air, has a beneficial action and played a part in allowing the patient to overcome the infection raging within his body.

Today, at long last, as more and more micro-organisms become resistant to antibiotics, and as more and more viruses are discovered against which no known antibiotics are effective, all but the most biased of research workers are beginning to admit that perhaps climatic conditions may play a part in causing, preventing, and curing infections of the body. Granted that those who look upon themselves as the élite of the medical research world are still insisting on remaining within their ivory towers and studying the defence mechanisms of the body to such good (or ill) effect that few but themselves can understand the resulting formulae, to few of which would Euclid have been able to subscribe Q.E.D. (Quod Erat Demonstrandum, or, in the schoolboy slang of my day: Quite Easily Done).

The trouble about biometeorology, to give it its formal Sunday name, as has already been noted, is that so many different factors are involved, such as temperature, humidity, barometric pressure, and their permutations and combinations on various fronts. To analyse the climatic conditions pertaining at any one time is tempting, indeed essential, but the unravelling of the Gordian knot is often impossible in our present state of knowledge.

Typical of the problems facing the observant doctor is that presented by the superintendent of a tuberculosis sanatorium some fifty years ago, who noted that his patients were liable to have haemoptyses (spitting up of blood) under two sets of conditions, best described in his own words. 'This was most frequent during an atmospheric condition of unresolved thunder – that is to say, heavy oppressive "headachey" weather. An actual thunder-storm did not do the same thing. The other condition was that of unresolved snow – that is to say, heavy snow clouds overhead but none falling. During actual falls of snow the symptom did not show itself.' It may well be that there were other meteorological factors with which the bleeding was associated, but obviously the doctor in question had the naturalist's approach to the problem, which is the basis of all sound medical practice.

Such anecdotal reports, as the modern medical statistician (who as often as not has seldom dealt with patients since he qualified) rather superciliously refers to them, must, let it be admitted, be handled with care, but two from the Orient, both dealing with plague, are of more than passing interest. One goes back to the devastating outbreak of plague in Manchuria in 1910–11 with its terrifying death-roll, due mainly to pneumonic plague, or plague pneumonia, the most fatal form of the disease. In this type of plague the *Bacillus pestis*, the causative organism, is spread by the patient coughing it up. In the intense cold of the Manchurian winter, during which the epidemic occurred, the exhaled, contaminated breath of the patients became visible due to the rapid condensation of its moisture content. Under these conditions of low temperature and condensing moisture the bacilli survived and were able to infect the other inhabitants of the poorly ventilated dwellings in which sick and healthy alike were lodged. By contrast, in India pneumonic plague was relatively rare, because, in the hot climate there, the droplets coughed out by the patients, and containing the bacilli, quickly dried and the bacilli were unable to survive.

'Dispersions', it is reported, 'in the air of other bacteria were found to be similarly affected. Thus, factors coming under the heading of weather were, for the first time, conclusively shown to have a possible effect on the ability of an agent responsible for an air-borne infection to remain infective and dangerous.' To which may be appended a comment from the original report: 'In other pneumonias . . . it is not unlikely that the dosage and virulence of the inhaled bacilli and the susceptibility of the host are factors of far greater importance than in plague pneumonia; hence the influence of atmospheric temperature in their spread would be more or less obscured by the other factors.'

Some sixty years later a United States report noted that in Vietnam plague in rats and man is inversely proportional to rainfall. The significance of this is that plague is primarily a disease of rats, among which it is spread by fleas. When these fleas are unable to find their natural hosts they patronise man and infect him with plague. To explain this relationship between rainfall and plague, the author of the report advances three suggestions. One is that when the fleas left the host rat in the rainy season they were trapped in the mud which formed in the rat burrow, rat-runs or feeding areas. The second is that during the monsoon the fleas are more liable to infection – and fleas, just like man, are afflicted by viruses and the like. The third is that adult fleas do not emerge from wet cocoons. In other words, the effect of climate in this instance is indirect rather than direct.

These two reports are typical examples of how, directly or indirectly, climate can play a part in enhancing, or diminishing, our protective measures against infection. By and large, the general consensus of opinion seems to be that temperature plays an important part. Typical of the evidence in favour of this is a report on the incidence of broncho-pneumonia in infants under two years of age in London in the sixteen years preceding the outbreak of the

1939–45 War, by two of the most distinguished London pathologists of their day. This showed a close association between the weekly mortality, not only of infants, but also of elderly folk over fifty-five years of age, from broncho-pneumonia, and the temperature twelve to fourteen days earlier. These findings, they comment, 'strengthen evidence that short spells of low temperature greatly raise the incidence of broncho-pneumonia in infants . . . The mortality of elderly persons over 55 years of age from broncho-pneumonia is also closely associated with temperature.'

To explain how this adverse effect is achieved, they suggest that 'adverse seasonal conditions may depress the resistance of the host to infection by causing a general deterioration in immunological defence mechanisms.' To which they add: 'There is now considerable evidence to support the clinical-statistical inference that exposure to low temperature has a detrimental effect upon the local defence mechanisms of the respiratory tract.' As an example of this they quote the case of a micro-organism known as *Haemophilus influenzae*. Confusingly, this organism has nothing to do with influenza (it received its misleading name under the mistaken impression that it was associated with the disease), but can cause serious lung trouble, particularly in people with chronic bronchitis. In the summer it is usually only found in the nose and throat, where it does no harm, but in later winter and early spring it tends to spread downwards into the lungs, where it can, and does, cause trouble.

One reason for this potentially dangerous migration is that adverse climatic conditions, including not only low temperature but also humidity, may affect the protecting cells lining the entrance to the lungs. Among these cells are some with what are called cilia, small lash-like processes which can maintain movement in the fluid moving over them in order to expel anything that may be damaging to the lungs, including micro-organisms. If these cilia, as a result of changes in temperature and/or humidity, are no longer able to function properly, microbes may be able to reach the lungs and cause trouble, such as bronchitis or pneumonia. In addition, in these adverse conditions microbes are able to slip in between the cells and get into the lungs in this way. There is also some evidence that these adverse climatic conditions can cut down the blood supply to the lining membranes of the air passage and thereby reduce their efficiency in resisting infection.

This is why there is so much to be said for bracing weather which stimulates the nasal and upper air passages thus causing an increased flow of blood to them, which ensures an adequate supply of oxygen and therefore a state of health. As evidence of this increased blood supply one can take the state of affairs when walking in a cold wind, which produces watering of the eyes and running of the nose. This has a further advantage because our tears contain a substance known as lysozyme, which was discovered by Sir Alexander Fleming, the discoverer of penicillin. Lysozyme kills bacteria, so that this free flow of tears and running of the nose not only washes out any offending bacteria but also kills off those not washed away. Here then is an example of cold being beneficial in protecting us from infection. It is also some consolation for those of us whose eyes water and nose runs so freely when we are out in a strong wind. It may be a nuisance, but it is helping to protect us from developing a cold, sore throat or the like. Nature is not so silly as we sometimes consider her to be.

The debit side of this balance sheet is summed up by the conclusions of the London pathologists' report. 'Their incompletely developed control of body temperature renders infants particularly vulnerable to adverse conditions, and it seems probable that any chilling of their bodies would lower the efficiency of the defence mechanisms of their respiratory tracts. Under these conditions, bacteria that are normal inhabitants of the nasopharynx [i.e. nose and throat] progressively extend their area of colonization until they gain access to the smaller bronchi and bronchioles [i.e. smaller air passages of the lungs] and there set up foci of broncho-pneumonia.'

A United States study of 'the climatic factor in precipitating acute tonsillitis in children' found that acute tonsillitis most often occurred in the wake of a cold front, or polar air mass, a time when air temperature falls, the barometric pressure rises and there is lessened humidity. This, it is claimed, affects the efficiency of the lining membrane of the nose and throat, sometimes after an interval of a few hours up to a day or two, and then allows any lurking micro-organisms to gain entry to the body and cause inflammation of the tonsils. This lowering of the resistance of the protective membrane of the nose and throat is partly produced by spasm of the blood-vessels which in turn results in a lack of oxygen. The effect of cold, however, it is noted, is only one of several meteorological factors. Lack of sunshine, change of barometric pressure, change in humidity and increased wind velocity are other factors that also accompany such a cold front and undoubtedly play a part in evoking a lowered local resistance to infection.

The position is further complicated, it has been pointed out, by the fact that meteorologically 'the population is constantly swinging from a phase where vascular spasm is enhanced to one where vascular dilatation is augmented, or vice-versa. The condition is one of constant flux in practically every physiological and biological balance. In the human being we deal with a continuous rhythm, of increasing and decreasing resistance from hour to hour, from day to day, and from season to season.' A further complication is that 'environmental alterations (for example, cooling) that can be useful to one individual by increasing tone during the phase of vascular spasm, may, in the inadequate individual, lessen resistance because of increasing fatigue.' All of which demonstrates the urgent need for research workers to descend from their ivory-tower concentration on antibiotics and the like, and turn their attention to the vagaries of the weather and its effect on the body's resistance to infection.

Typical of the research work on the effect of thermal stress in facilitating infection that needs to be followed up is that done some fifteen years ago in the Netherlands. This showed that after cooling the hand at 50° F. (10° C.) for two minutes, normal temperature was regained in six minutes in healthy subjects but took much longer in patients with a wide variety of illness, including the common cold. This failure to regain normal temperature was attributed to a failure of the normal thermoregulation (heat control) of the body. A further indication of the complexity of the problem is the finding that, in a 'cattery', exposure of the kittens to a double thermal stress while they were incubating a virus infection induced epidemics of the disease.

This 'double stress' is referred to in an interesting report from a Derbyshire general practitioner based on a study of 758 patients during the winter of 1970–1, who found that 'temperature fluctuation, particularly when repeated, was found to be the most significant factor, with school terms contributing markedly to the morbidity.' To which he adds the comment: 'The failure of the thermoregulation of the body, and more specifically of the nasal mucosa [lining membrane of the nose], in response to temperature stress is suggested as a possible mechanism which facilitates the development of virus to produce a common-cold infection.' 'It was natural', he added, 'that a single large fluctuation [in temperature] was less likely to give a "cold" increase than a double or multiple oscillation as in the case of the kittens.'

In this context it is of interest to note that a fellow-practitioner in Gloucestershire, on the basis of the records of 150 of his patients who volunteered to keep a diary record of their experience with the common cold over a period of five years, reported a close correlation of the incidence of colds with a fall in external temperature: for each 1° F. (0·50° C.) fall in external temperature there was a 1 per cent rise in the incidence of colds. To complete a trilogy of reports from England, one from the Public Health Laboratory Service, based on studies in London and Newcastle over four and six years, respectively, may be quoted. This revealed a 'mean negative correlation between the number of colds reported as starting on a given day and the mean outdoor day temperature . . . independent of the intercorrelation of tempera- ture and the other meteorological variables studied, that is, water-vapour pressure, relative humidity, difference between maximum day temperature and minimum night temperature, rain, hours of sunlight, atmospheric pollution, cyclonic or anticyclonic weather.' To this they add: 'Of these, only water-vapour pressure shows a small but perhaps significant independent association with colds. The correlation reaches a maximum value between the colds caught and the temperature difference, that is its fall below the expected value for the time of year, about three days before.' 'This time interval', it is said, 'is so close to the median interval between inoculation [that is, infection with the virus] and the development of symptoms as to suggest that some consequence of lowered external temperature exerts a direct influence on the transmission of infection.' If only we knew the answer to this secret, how much further forward we might be in dealing, not only with the so-called common cold, but also infection with any micro-organism.

Pending further investigation into this maze, which should be high on the priority list of the Medical Research Council, the Department of Health and Social Security and all those foundations subsidising medical research, there are two further aspects that deserve mention. One is the report from the Indian Army medical service, already referred to in chapter 5, that at high altitudes there is a decrease in disease due to viruses and bacteria, compared with the state of affairs at sea level. Follow-up of this finding showed that it was associated with an increase in the amount of what is known as immunoglobulin in those living at high altitudes [in this case, 12 000 to 18 000 feet (3700 to 5500 metres)] as compared with those living at sea level. This applied not only to the permanent inhabitants at high altitudes but also the troops when they were posted to those lofty heights. As immunoglobulins are among the important agents produced in the body to protect it against infection, this indicates yet another means whereby atmospheric conditions affect the incidence of diseases due to infection. How this protective mechanism is induced is still unknown.

The final factor for consideration is the part played by

atmospheric, or air, ions, which are discussed more fully in chapter 2. All that need be said here is that there is quite impressive evidence that negative air ions have a lethal action on micro-organisms. Conversely there is evidence that positive air ions may facilitate infection. This is a subject that has been largely ignored in Britain, but research work in the United States, Israel and elsewhere indicates that these ions may play a quite considerable part in the control of infectious diseases in both man and animals. Whether their artificial production has any therapeutic value is still *sub judice*, but undoubtedly they are deserving of much more attention than they have received in the past.

15

Climate and rheumatism

'Therefore the moon, the governess of floods,
Pale in her anger, washes all the air,
That rheumatic diseases do abound.'
A Midsummer Night's Dream

'Hark how the chairs and tables crack!
Old Betty's joints are on the rack;'

'When rheumatic people complain of more than ordinary
pains in the joints, it will rain.'

Whatever the clever scientists and modern doctors may think, the
public have no doubt about the association between climate and
rheumatism, as illustrated in these three examples of weather lore.
The sceptical scientist may, in the words of the old fairy tale, puff
and puff, but he will never blow this particular house down.
Indeed, one gets the impression that all but the most virulent critics
of the association have a sneaking feeling that folk lore is right and
wish they could find convincing evidence to support it. They may
be statistically suspicious of what they call anecdotal evidence but,
like it or not, they cannot resist quoting examples such as the
following two, taken from a report from the Mayo Clinic, for
long regarded as the *sanctum sanctorum* of American medicine.

'On one morning during early summer we were all pleased with the general sense of well being which prevailed among the patients with arthritis. The sun was shining brightly and there was not a cloud in the sky. Early in the afternoon one patient after another, twelve in all, began to call for some sort of relief for pain. This seemed remarkable since the sky was still clear, but later that afternoon an electrical storm suddenly appeared.' 'A 7-year-old girl with arthritis when asked if she ever suffered pain, replied: "Yes, whenever we have a storm my joints feel stiff and I feel sore all over; and after the storm has gone I feel pretty well again, but I am sometimes better before the rain stops".'

Perhaps the best summing up of the view of the more objective reviewers of the rheumatic scene is that of a former member of the staff of the Medical Research Council National Institute for Medical Research, which is given *in extenso* as it so admirably assesses the available evidence.

'Chronic rheumatic patients frequently relate certain types of symptoms to the weather, but their histories conform to no uniform pattern. Some appear to notice an increase in symptoms the day before a change of weather – the rheumatic "weather prophets"; others describe increased pain and stiffness in cold, damp, windy or thundery weather, respectively, and some even in hot weather . . . Medical climatologists believe that it is the suddenness and irregularity of changes of weather rather than the particular types of weather that are significant in relation to rheumatic symptoms. This climatic instability, which is characteristic of the temperate zone, is due to the passage of air masses of different origin and composition without any regular order or sequence. The physiological and pathological effects on man of the passage of polar and tropical air masses and the associated variations in atmospheric pressure, barometric pressure, wind, humidity and solar radiation were studied by Professor Petersen. He presented an astonishing array of charts showing biochemical rhythms in the body that appear to run parallel to weather changes. Petersen's work has not gone unchallenged [which is putting it mildly], but many of his biochemical results have subsequently been confirmed and his thesis may well prove to be sound.'

All of which was concisely epitomised by Professor G. E. Burch, the New Orleans authority on the effect of climate on the heart: 'Today it is well acknowledged that the natural history of some diseases, such as bronchial asthma, chronic bronchitis, and rheumatoid arthritis, is often modified by fluctuations in the weather and climate.' On the other hand, the ambivalent attitude of so many modern rheumatologists is exemplified in the answer of the anonymous consultant of the *British Medical Journal* to a reader's query as to whether 'there is any firm evidence that geographical location or climate have any effect on the development and progress of "rheumatic" or "arthritic" processes.' The gist of the answer was: 'Geography and climate do not exert a strong influence on rheumatic conditions' but, it was added, 'most arthritics find their symptoms more tolerable in dry, moderate heat, but a few prefer the cold.' An admirable example of the Mr Facing-both-ways attitude, or sitting on the fence.

Perhaps the most detailed study of the general picture is the Mayo Clinic report already quoted. This was based on a study of 367 patients with arthritis seen during the course of one year. For only 7 per cent of the time was there no correlation between barometric pressure and the degree of pain. When the severity of the pain was not in accord with changes in barometric pressure, this was almost invariably related to the presence of storms or marked changes in the weather. For almost 90 per cent of the year, the presence of a storm was associated with increased pain. So far as humidity was concerned, the authors of the report were unable to show any definite correlation with pain. Their impression was that 'it would seem that humidity alone is not an important factor', 'but it is possible,' they add, that 'further work may show that in combination with other factors it is of some significance.'

Further work has supported this point of view, such as that carried out in the controlled-climate chamber, or Climatron, designed and built at the University of Pennsylvania, Philadelphia, which permits the manipulation of temperature, humidity, barometric pressure, rate of air flow and ion concentration. This showed that 'falling barometric pressure with rising humidity has a nearly constant detrimental effect on rheumatoid arthritis and osteoarthrosis, whereas no single variation to climate can produce such an effect.' A word of warning, however, must be repeated here as to the possible fallacy of such experiments in climatic chambers. The weather is such a complex of factors that attempting to analyse any one factor, such as humidity, for example, may be misleading if interpreted in isolation. It may well be a basically sound approach, but the results must be interpreted with caution. So far as barometric pressure and rheumatic pains are concerned, it is of interest that it has often been observed that divers subject to such pains obtain relief while diving – that is, under pressure, and this relief continues for some time after the divers have surfaced and been decompressed.

The unsolved mystery is how these various meteorological changes produce their effect. One suggestion is that patients with rheumatoid arthritis have peripheral blood-vessels that are easily constricted. This high vascular tone, with the increased spastic response to any adverse factor, such as cold, by over-constricting and thereby depriving the joints of an adequate supply of blood might well explain why such people are liable to develop the disease. All of us respond to cold by developing cold hands, which is a defence mechanism to restrict the amount of heat we lose and so help to maintain the temperature of the body, and it is produced by constriction of the blood-vessels in the skin. In those who develop rheumatoid arthritis the constriction is overdone and slow to relax, thereby depriving the tissues of an adequate blood supply, with consequent degenerative changes.

Such a state of affairs would explain quite a number of the

features of rheumatoid arthritis, as, for example, the cold hands and feet, of which they complain so bitterly. It would also explain why the disease is more common in cold countries and much less common in warm zones where there is not the same continual stimulation of low temperatures to keep the blood-vessels constricted. It could also be the explanation of why so many of the commonly quoted precipitating factors in the disease, such as cold and damp, mental and physical strain, and infection, produce their effects. All are known to be capable of producing constriction of the blood-vessels. Further, it would explain why some patients, if not all, obtain benefit from a constant dry, warm atmosphere. Incidentally, it is an indication of why they should keep themselves warmly clothed and avoid being chilled.

Indirect confirmation of this possible causative factor comes from a Swedish report describing how seven patients were kept for long periods in a climatic chamber, or laboratory, at the equivalent of a relatively warm dry tropical climate. In all of them the peripheral circulation was improved, and constricted blood-vessels dilated with a raising of the temperature of the skin, especially of the hands and feet. The ultimate result was that four of the patients were relieved of their symptoms and returned to work. Two improved but relapsed quickly after completing the course, whilst one did not complete the course.

Another approach to the problem was mediated in Canada, where it was shown that on exposure to zero or subzero temperatures the knee joint of cats fell to a lower temperature than the rest of the body, and that this low joint temperature was accompanied by increased stiffness of the joint. This led on to a study of the speed of bending of the index finger before and after exposure to cold, which confirmed that 'on exposure to cold the maximum speed with which a joint can be moved decreases.' Studies of the joint fluid showed that as the temperature of the joint fell the fluid became more viscid or sticky due to an increase in the amount of a substance known as mucin. This increased viscosity due to cold, it was concluded, explained the loss of speed of movement of the joint. It would explain why, in rheumatic subjects, the joints stiffen up in cold weather.

One more approach to the problem is worthy of mention. It is known that in inflammatory conditions such as rheumatoid arthritis there is a deposition in the effected joints of a substance known as fibrin. Persistence of this substance might well be an important factor in rheumatoid arthritis. Should this be a correct hypothesis, then anything that removes the fibrin should be of help in arresting, if not curing, the condition. Working on this idea, a group of investigators in this country gave a series of patients with rheumatoid arthritis a drug, known as phenformin, which is known to facilitate the removal of fibrin. Of the sixteen patients given the drug, twelve responded satisfactorily. Not satisfied with these results, the investigators carried out a further trial with twenty patients, giving them two drugs (one of them phenformin) which speed up the removal of fibrin. Twelve of this group of patients had what is described as 'worth-while' improvement.

As no follow-up of these two reports has appeared, it may well be that later results did not confirm the original findings, but they are worthy of note as indicating the intricacy of the rheumatic problem. Their relevance to the climatic approach is that there is evidence of an association between climate and clotting of the blood, and fibrin is one of the factors involved in this complex process. Thus there is evidence of increased fibrinolytic activity (the process whereby fibrin is disposed of in the body) at high altitudes, which may be one reason why there is less arthritis at high altitudes than at sea level. Two other factors may play a part here. One is that there are reports purporting to show that at high altitudes there is an increased production of the cortisone-like substances that are known to have a beneficial effect in rheumatoid arthritis. The other is that at high altitudes there is an increased production of immunoglobulins, an integral part of our defence mechanisms against infection, and this may be a protective factor if, as is still a possibility, rheumatoid arthritis is due to some obscure infection with a micro-organism.

In *Rheumatism in Populations*, the most recent and authoritative review of the subject, Dr J. S. Lawrence points out that rheumatic complaints are a more important cause of incapacity in Northern European countries such as Norway, Sweden and the United Kingdom than in Central Europe or the U.S.A. There is even an indication that such climatic differences as exist between the north and the south of England have an appreciable effect. Thus studies carried out in Leigh in Lancashire, Wensleydale in Yorkshire, and Watford in Hertfordshire, indicated that approximately twice as many persons lost time off work from rheumatic complaints in Leigh and Wensleydale than in Watford. These studies also suggested that 'incapacity fitted most closely the hours of sunshine and appeared to be related to solar radiation rather than to temperature.' An extension of these studies to Jamaica showed that rheumatic complaints as a whole were less common in Jamaica, loss of work from rheumatic complaints being less than half as frequent in Jamaica than in the English studies. Osteoarthrosis, on the other hand, was just as frequent in Jamaica as in England, but Jamaicans had less symptoms from it than their counterparts in the north of England.

His summing up is that, 'although there is no evidence that climate plays a part in the etiology [causation] of rheumatoid arthritis, there are indications that the weather may affect the activity of the arthritic process.' This is in line with his Manchester colleague, Professor J. H. Kelgren, according to whom, 'the climatic environment has not been shown to influence the prevalence and severity of joint disease, but it does appear to influence the complaint threshold.' Thus, he notes, 'pain and disability are greater than expected in men working in a cold, wet environment and less than expected in those working in a hot, dry environment.' 'This', he graciously concedes, 'is in accordance with popular belief.' His conclusion is that a 'genetically determined predisposition and environmental factors are of roughly equal importance in the causation of most rheumatic diseases.' Although he does not specifically include climate among his 'environmental factors', all the available evidence suggests, if not indicates, that this is a perfectly justifiable inclusion.

A further point brought out by Professor Kelgren and his colleagues is that rheumatic patients tend to be hypersensitive to pain, and that this sensitivity is influenced by quite small changes in the temperature of the affected tissues, whether muscles or joints. As cooling occurs more easily in a wet than a dry atmosphere, this might explain the difference found by Professor Kelgren between men working in dry and wet atmospheres. Or, in Dr Lawrence's words: 'It may be supposed that in a warm climate local or referred hyperalgesia [i.e. hypersensitivity to pain] occurs but is not sufficient to give rise to spontaneous pain. When tissue temperature falls from reduction of air temperature or diminished solar radiation, or from the influence of increased humidity, spontaneous pain arises.'

It takes time, however, to lower the temperature of the deeper tissues of the body, and, as Dr L. G. C. Pugh has pointed out, 'the onset of pain in response to cold is often too rapid to be explained on this basis. Some patients, for instance, complain of pain coming on immediately on getting into a cold bed or going out on a cold day. In such cases the rapid onset of pain suggests a reflex nervous mechanism.' 'A possible explanation' he puts forward is that 'cold-sensitive subjects respond to cold stimuli, applied to a wide area of the body surface, with muscle tension more readily than average subjects, and that this may exaggerate any tendency to muscle spasm [a painful process as anyone knows who has had cramp in the leg] in regions giving rise to rheumatic symptoms.' It is interesting how similar this suggestion is to one put forward by a distinguished predecessor at the National Institute for Medical Research half a century earlier, Sir Leonard Hill: 'Rheumatic pains so notoriously increased by a change to cold damp weather, may be due to increased tension in nerve sheaths, nerve endings etc., induced by lessened evaporation or by shrinkage due to cold.'

One final factor in the intriguing, if still mystifying, problem of climate and rheumatism. That is that a fall in barometric pressure and increasing humidity, either separately or together, may lead to a retention of water in the body, and that this may be responsible for rheumatic aches and pains. The suggested rationale here is that normally where these two climatic conditions are accompanied by an increased output of urine, the extra fluid involved being extruded from the body cells into the bloodstream because, of course, the volume of circulating blood must be maintained if the body is to continue to function normally. The cells of diseased tissue, however, such as rheumatic tissue, are not as permeable as healthy cells and therefore retain their fluid. This in turn results in a relatively higher pressure in these rheumatic cells compared with the surrounding healthy cells. It is this gradient, or difference, of pressure which is said to lead to pain and the characteristic swelling of the diseased part.

Rheumatism may not be a killing disease, but it is a devastatingly crippling one, to which much too little attention has ever been devoted. The sooner this situation is remedied the better, and it is clear from a perusal of the available information that one of the first problems to be tackled is that of climate and rheumatism. Unfortunately the powers that be tend to look down their scientific noses at what they obviously consider to be a plebeian subject beneath their dignity. The truth is that they are avoiding it because it is too complex and does not lend itself to investigation by expensive electronic apparatus and instruments in chromium-plated laboratories.

It is up to the large rheumatic element in the community to correct this unbalanced outlook and insist on more money being spent on elucidating the climatic problem of their disease. Meanwhile they should take avoiding action by living, whenever possible, in warm, dry climes, particularly during the winter, wearing comfortable warm clothing, living in centrally heated houses, and keeping themselves as generally fit as possible. This last is as important as anything because there is little, if any, doubt that any lowering of the defence mechanisms of the body leads to exacerbations of the rheumatic process – whatever that may be.

16

Climate and migraine

Thursday 18 May I find myself a very fairly reliable means of prognosticating blizzards for I almost invariably get a sort of migraine headache 10 or 12 hours before the blizzard begins. Today was the third time and again it was right.

Sunday 18 June 1911 1st Sunday after Trinity. Again had a blizzard headache in the night and though it was dead calm when we were at breakfast the blizzard came on with a whoop after a blow all day.

These two excerpts from the diary kept by Dr Edward Wilson of the ill-fated *Terra Nova* expedition to the Antarctic, in which both Captain Scott and Dr Wilson perished on 21 March 1912, are classical examples of a long recognised association between climate, particularly wind, and migraine. In the characteristically brisk language of Mr Peter Wilson, the honorary secretary of the British Migraine Association, in a recent letter to me: 'High winds, of course, affect us all, and in Cape Town when the wind blows there for weeks on end the consumption of aspirin and the murder rate go sky high. Almost every Miggie [his nickname for migrainous subjects, of which he is one himself] is highly susceptible to high winds, probably because they are a source of irritation but even when indoors the headaches still occur.'

The extent of this association and its possible *modus operandi* were cogently reviewed in a report in 1974 from the Department of Applied Pharmacology and Bioclimatology of Hebrew University, Jerusalem, which Dr F. G. Sulman, the senior author of the report, summarised in *Hemicrania*, the journal of the Migraine Trust. 'Hot winds of ill repute in all parts of the world', he noted, 'affect mental and physical well-being and may constitute a factor in provoking migraine in weather-sensitive patients. Such winds are known by various terms, e.g. the Santa Ana of Southern California; the desert winds of Arizona; the Argentine Zonda; the Sirocco and Tramontana of the Mediterranean littoral; the Meltemia of Greece (referred to as *Etesiae* by Homer); the Maltesian Xlokk; the Chamsin or Sharkiye of the Arab countries; the Sharav of the Old Testament, which still scourges Israel; the Foehn of Switzerland, Southern Germany and Austria, well known to the Romans as *Favonius*; the Autun of France; the northern winds of Melbourne; the Thar winds of India; the Chinook of Canada; the Gonding and Koembang of Java and the Bohoroh of Sumatra. These weather conditions are notorious for their association with headache, depression, discomfort, irritability and the exacerbation of respiratory conditions in certain patients, and the existence of a variety of migraine due to some meteorological changes is mentioned in monographs dealing with migraine.'

Such was the background to the investigation initiated by Dr Sulman and his colleagues, in which they studied some 500 patients who were susceptible to the Sharav. A preliminary study revealed that what they describe as the 'climatic heat-stress' induced by the Sharav was accompanied by three meteorological changes: (i) a decrease in relative humidity to values below 25 to 30 per cent; (ii) an increase in temperature of up to 27° F. (15° C.) above the average for the time of year; (iii) the presence of eastern air currents (desert winds). These created a high level of electricity similar to a thunderstorm and characterised by the presence of positive air ions (up to 4000, as opposed to the normal 1100 to 1200 per cubic centimetre). 'These meteorological phenomena', it was found, 'arrive one or two days before the weather-front, and sensitive subjects are true "weather prophets", and migrainous headaches resulted in 20 to 40 per cent of those affected.'

Their most interesting finding in what is quite a complex situation, which is being deliberately simplified (though not falsified) for the sake of brevity and lay understanding, was that in migrainous subjects, amongst others, these meteorological changes were accompanied by an increased output of a neurohormone known as serotonin. The significance of this is that serotonin contracts the peripheral blood-vessels, including those of the lining membrane of the brain, and thereby induces a migrainous attack. It is because they antagonise, or neutralise, this action of serotonin that drugs such as ergotamine and methysergide are so effective in alleviating or preventing the headaches of migraine.

Inevitably the association of migraine with a high positive air-ion level suggested that treatment with artificially produced negative air ions, which are known to antagonise positive air ions, might be helpful. The preliminary results of such treatment suggested that it might be of value, but the fact that little more has been heard of it indicates that it has proved of little help, or, possibly, that the results were not as satisfactory as with standard anti-serotonin drugs. What is of interest, and it is worthy of note, is that at the turn of the present century the suggestion was advanced that migraine, amongst other conditions, might depend on changes in atmospheric potential and a high level of positive air ions. Another example of there being 'no new thing under the sun'. From the practical point of view the interest of this observation is that here we have a clear-cut explanation of the association of certain climatic factors and migraine.

The only other relatively recent study of climate and migraine comes from Aberdeen, based on a study of fifty-six subjects during a six-month, winter and spring period (November to May). This shows that the percentage of severe migrainous attacks was significantly increased during days when there were more than two hours of sunshine and when this gave rise to dazzle in combination with snow. Atmospheric cooling was reported as a causative or aggravating factor by seven and in 1·2 per cent of recorded attacks. A low atmospheric pressure recorded at noon tended to be associated with significantly less frequent attacks, and there was a trend towards an increase in frequency of attacks when the atmospheric pressure was rising, as was also the case with low relative humidity. This association of severe attacks under conditions of low relative humidity, it is suggested, 'may be associated with an increase in positive ionization as described by Sulman and his colleagues before the dry wind known as Sharav.'

Over half the patients recorded attacks considered to be due to recognisable weather conditions, though recorded attacks due to the weather constituted only 2·5 per cent of all attacks, compared, for example, with fatigue which was considered responsible for a quarter of all attacks, and menstruation which was associated with 6 per cent of attacks, whilst one half of the attacks had no recognisable cause. Few of the volunteers mentioned thunder-storms as a precipitant of migraine, but this might be partially explained by the fact that the presence of the Cairngorms protects Aberdeen from such electrical disturbances, and it is noted that letters from sufferers in other parts of the country mentioned thunderstorms as a cause. Finally, it is reported that those who suspected an association between weather conditions and migraine considered that these were 'aggravating rather than causative.' This, it is considered, is borne out by the fact that weather conditions with an effect on migraine influenced the severity rather than the frequency of attacks.

All of which suggests that there is some association between climate and migraine, a view that is shared by Dr Macdonald Critchley, the grand old man of British neurology, who has made a special study of migraine. Is it possible that migrainous subjects are among the 'weather-sensitive' section of the community? Whatever the answer, it would appear that the problem is worth further study, if only to allow the victims of this devastating affliction to forecast when an attack is impending. This is much more important than it may sound because, in Mr Peter Wilson's pleasantly plain language, 'time is the essence and don't I know it. I lost two pounds last week in a puking exercise just because I waited five minutes longer'. Might it not be worth while the British Migraine Association and the Migraine Trust joining forces to issue a national questionnaire spread over a year to discover the response of British migrainous subjects to the vagaries of our climate?

17

Climate and cancer

'This phenomenon of the clinical manifestation of recurrence of an apparently healed malignant tumour, within a year and sometimes within a few months after a bereavement, has been observed by a number of clinicians . . .

'I have often felt that malignant tumours tend to respond badly to treatment in conscientious patients whom one feels can be described as unusually good citizens . . .

'I have often noticed characteristic types of personality in patients with malignant disease, especially carcinoma of the lung, carcinoma of the rectum and chronic myeloid leukaemia . . .

'I have often tried in talking to patients about their illness to lead them to a more peaceful permanent state of mind in the hope that the neoplastic disease will respond better to treatment and be less likely to recur.'

These quotations from the opening address by the then Regius Professor of Physic in Cambridge University, one of the leading radiotherapists of his generation, to the Third International Conference of the International Psychosomatic Cancer Study Group in 1963, are not as irrelevant to the subject of this chapter as might appear because, as Dr W. S. Tromp, Head of the Biometeorological Research Centre at Leiden, who has written more extensively and stimulatingly on the subject of climate and disease than almost anyone else, pointed out in his paper to the Conference, 'both during psychological and meteorological stresses a considerable disturbance in hormonal balance can be observed.' 'As it is almost certain that in most neoplastic diseases', he continued, 'serious disturbances may play a very important part, either in the initial development or during the later stages of the disease, it seems possible, at least on theoretical grounds, that meteorological stresses could be able to affect neoplastic diseases.'

In a subsequent report he developed this theme, laying emphasis on the disturbance of heat control, or thermoregulation, induced by cold and how this affects various brain centres. 'Many physiological studies have shown that each of the centres described are affected both by psychological and meteorological stresses.' 'Both types of stress', he adds, 'trigger the same physiological mechanisms in the human body and therefore there is no reason to assume that meteorological stresses would not affect neoplastic diseases in a similar way as in the case of psychological stress.'

How the thermoregulatory efficiency of the cancer patient is affected was impressively shown in an investigation he carried out on fifty patients with cancer at the cancer clinic of the Antoni van Leeuwenhoek-huis, Amsterdam. All responded badly to a standard test of thermoregulation, as compared with normal individuals, the response being particularly poor in advanced inoperable cases. Conversely, after removal of the breast in cases of cancer of the breast the response improved rapidly. The same response to treatment was noted in cases of cancer of the cervix of the uterus. 'After the cancer patient had been operated on, and completely recovered', it is recorded, 'the thermoregulation curves are almost similar to those of normals.' His final conclusion is that 'it seems most likely that extreme meteorological stresses could seriously affect the state of health of the cancer patient through hypothalamic stresses.' The hypothalamus, it may be interpolated, is that part of the brain that exerts control over many of the hormones of the body.

In animal experiments he reports that at the same clinic in a strain of mice known for its high incidence of cancer of the breast, in mice born in the winter the incidence of cancer was 12 per cent higher than in those born in the summer. And he reports a comparable finding in over 700 rats in which tumours were implanted over a two-year period. The number of rats in which the tumour 'took', or grew, increased during the approach of cold fronts and dropped again after the front had passed. This effect was most marked when the meteorological stimulus took place one or two days after the tumour had been implanted.

Conversely, it is known that high temperatures have a relatively retarding effect on the growth of tumours. This has been demonstrated in both animals and human beings. There is also experimental evidence that rapidly growing implanted tumours in rats and mice show a greatly diminished rate of growth during prolonged exposure, say, for a fortnight, to low pressures of oxygen such as exist at altitudes of around 20 000 feet (6500 metres). The author of one of these reports, however, cautiously adds a note to the effect that 'so far as these experiments go there is no evidence that alterations – within the limits of safety – of oxygen pressure are by themselves of therapeutic value.' Exposure to high pressures of oxygen, it was reported, produced no effect on the tumours. On the other hand, for a time patients receiving radiotherapy for the treatment of cancer were given their treatment at a high concentration of oxygen in the belief that this increased oxygen concentration improved the benefit derived from the radiotherapy. This observation, however, has not stood up to the test of time.

The snag is that, when it is attempted to translate these experimental observations into terms of cancer in man, the picture is far from clear. Thus, according to one United States report, based on the findings in 163 large cities in 1949–51, and 50 countries in 1959–63, 'chilling effect of wind and low temperature combined showed a highly significant statistical relationship to mortality from cancer of the lung' but, it is added, 'though it appears likely that environmental chilling may be a contributory factor in malignancy death rates, the relationship is not a simple one.' On the other hand, a report published in 1977, comparing deaths over a four-year period in Pittsburgh, Pennsylvania, and Birmingham, Alabama, indicated that the weather 'affected little mortality from cancer.'

In contrast is a series of reports from the Statistics Unit of the Imperial Cancer Research Fund. According to the last of these, a highly significant correlation was found between the death rate from cancer of the breast in women in thirty-three countries and the environmental temperature, the death rate rising with a rise in temperature. The plaintive note, however, is added: 'This provides further confirmation of the still completely unexplained relation between neoplasms of the breast and environmental temperature.' A follow-up report from the same laboratories indicated that induced breast tumours in mice occurred earlier and in more animals when they were exposed to high temperatures.

Another approach to the problem is based on a study of the seasonal incidence of tumours. This is a maze of frightening complexity, but a report from the Medical Research Council Social Medicine Research Unit usefully clarifies some of the most salient features. The two definite facts that emerge are that children showed the largest and most consistent summer increase in deaths from malignant disease, and that at all ages the maximum mortality from acute leukaemia was in July. On the latter finding the comment is made that 'this distribution is very unlikely to be due to chance, and is one of the pieces of evidence that makes it difficult to account for the observations except in terms of a real effect of the summer on the host/disease relationship.' A somewhat heavy way of saying that there was no doubt about the facts. What makes this finding more plausible or explicable is the current view that leukaemia is a virus infection, and it is known that various meteorological factors have an adverse effect on viruses and also affect the defence mechanism of the body against infection.

The position with regard to other tumours is nothing like so clear. There is some evidence that deaths from cancer of the testis is more common in the summer, as are the number of women first reporting with cancer of the breast, and the number of first hospital visits for cancer of the rectum. As is pointed out, however, 'other factors may come into play such as a woman being more likely to notice a lump in the breast in early summer because of the change to lighter (and probably new) clothing.' The cautious conclusion reached is that, 'while these data are compatible with the hypothesis that early cases of a variety of tumours present more often in summer than in winter, they do not prove this.' If the hypothesis is true, and it clearly cannot be dismissed out of hand, the following further comment is worthy of note. 'Apart from a few, malignant tumours are not exposed to the outside environment. They have no information concerning the changing seasons except for changes in the patient's internal state. Thus it appears that there exists a system in the human being which has the properties of changing with the seasons, and affecting the progress of some malignant diseases.' To which is added the sobering comment that 'we are quite ignorant of the mechanism which produces this effect,' but, it is added, 'the adrenal hormones are obvious candidates.'

There – with one exception, to be discussed in a moment – we must leave the problem. All the evidence suggests that there is some relation between climate and cancer, but proof is lacking. Whether such proof can be obtained is problematical, but the general impression left on the mind of the impartial observer is that, as in so many aspects of climate and disease, the powers that be have been sadly lacking in the attention they have devoted to the problem. Granted that it is a hard nut to crack but that is no excuse for ignoring it. Rather should it be a stimulus to the research worker who, in the past at least, welcomed a challenge and went all out to 'solve the insoluble'. Today, alas, priority is all too often given to the line of research that will produce the quickest results and the maximal number of published articles to be added to the *curriculum vitae* of the applicant for a job.

The final word, however, can be more precise and practical. There is one form of cancer that is undoubtedly due to climate and that is cancer of the skin. As noted in chapter 8, this is due to over-exposure to a certain range of the ultra-violet rays of the sun. This is not a problem we are faced with in the British Isles, but it is a very real problem in countries such as Australia, where a white population lives in a climate with a large amount of sunshine. There, where sun-bathing with the minimum of clothing required by the law (and that couldn't be much more minuscular) the incidence is quite high. It is the blonde, fair-haired, blue-eyed, so-called Celtic type who is most prone to it. Anyone of this make-up should therefore be reticent in over-exposing him- or her-self to the sun's rays. If, and when, they do, initial exposure should be gradual, so as to allow the maximal tanning of the skin. This will not guarantee protection from cancerous degeneration of the skin, but it will reduce the risk.

An interesting aspect of this problem is the recent report (1978) from U.S.A., indicating an association between sun spots and cancer of the skin. Similar reports have come from Finland. Sunspot activity, which occurs in cycles of eight to eleven years, involves the arousal of powerful magnetic fields. These influence the entrance of cosmic rays into the stratosphere, resulting in an increase in the rate of destruction of the ozone which shields us against excessive exposure to the cancer-inducing ultra-violet irradiation (see chapter 9).

For those who tan for aesthetic reasons, the wise rule is, once this has been achieved, to cut down exposure to the sun by, for example, wearing a straw hat with a wide brim so as to provide a fair degree of protection, and a modicum – not a minimum – of clothing. So far as the ladies are concerned, such protection of the nude skin can be as aesthetically pleasing, and as sexually attractive – if not more so – than the near-nude state so widely sported today. For the male who wishes to be elegant, it takes a lot to beat the old-fashioned panama. The topi may not be necessary as a protection against 'sunstroke', but something comparable should be worn to provide some protection from cancer of the skin which may respond readily to treatment if dealt with in time, but is an unnecessary hazard to life.

18

Climate and the psyche

Discussing the weather is said to be one of our national traits, but the belief in the association of climate and our emotions knows no national bounds. All down the ages poets and philosophers have waxed eloquent on the subject, and innumerable are the theories evoked by clever doctors as to how and why this occurs. Swinburne's reference to 'sad or singing weather' is but an echo of, for example, Virgil in the first book of his *Georgics*:

> 'Thus when the changeful temper of the skies
> The rare condenses, the dense rarefies,
> New motions on the altered air impressed
> New images and passions fill the breast;'

or Montaigne with his comment that

> 'The minds of men do in the weather share,
> Dark or serene as the day's foul or fair.'

All of which was amplified from personal experience by Burton in his *Anatomy of Melancholy*: 'Weather works on all in different degrees, but most on those who are disposed to melancholy. The devil himself seems to take the opportunity of foul and tempestuous weather to agitate our spirits and humours in our bodies tossed with tempestuous winds and storms.'

Which is simply a pleasingly poetic way of saying what

A Change of Air

Professor G. E. Burch, of New Orleans, the outstanding investigator of the effect of climate on the heart, has epitomised in our own generation. 'It is well known that man is affected mentally and physically by climate and weather and that some diseases are almost totally under the influence of the weather . . . A sudden fall in barometric pressure tends to be associated with mental depression. Crises of violence, traffic and industrial accidents, suicides and certain diseases seem to occur most often after a decline in barometric pressure. Hot and humid weather is also associated with depression and lassitude. Crime rates are highest in the summer. Most revolutions occur during the summer as is evidenced by the fact that Independence Day and Bastille Day are both in July.'

This last thought is an interesting one, but whether it is as true today, when revolutions seem to be two a penny, is another matter. If the climatic correlation is not as close as it might be, perhaps this is because so many more of us are living in man-controlled micro-climates which protect us from the full onslaught of the macro-climate, whether this be extreme heat or cold. To have a comfortable cool home to return to and cool off, psychologically as well as physically, may be an excellent way of reducing emotional pressures before they reach exploding point.

Be all that as it may, before turning to the evidence to back up the claim that the association is causative rather than coincidental, a salutary tale from the Orient is worthy of note, as recorded in the Proceedings of the Royal Meteorological Society in the 1930s by a member who had spent many years in China. 'On occasions at Shanghai', he writes, 'the Chinese behaved strangely in the fast and heavy traffic of the Nangking Road. This strange behaviour took two distinct forms which did not merge one into the other nor with the normal. The two states were absolutely distinct and unmistakable. One was an abnormality of lethargy; the other an abnormality of excitement. In the first, men, women and children sauntered slowly across the street, looking neither to the right nor the left, with a complete disregard of motor-cars. It was not a manifestation of bravado but one of superb indifference to danger. In the other, small boys dashed in and out of the traffic and doubled back like rabbits; old women put their heads down and fluttered across like hens; and rickshaw men bounded along at extra speed, swerving to the right and left in an ecstasy of life and vigour. One or other of these phenomena occurred at intervals of perhaps a fortnight or perhaps a month.'

Unable to correlate these curious oddities of behaviour – so reminiscent of a Monsieur Hulot film – with any specific meteorological phenomenon, phases of the moon or sunspots, the conclusion is reached that 'this strange behaviour was due to some unknown stimulus in the climate; something of the sort that causes excitement among the dragon-flies when a typhoon is approaching.' An intriguing postscript records that the author 'sought the same phenomena on the Continent', but 'only in Paris did he find something analogous. It is well known there that on occasion, and collectively, the taxi drivers have wild orgies in their art of skilful, reckless driving.'

Before passing to the more substantive, if plebeian, aspects of the subject, the reference to the phases of the moon may be taken up. The association between the moon and mental illness is as old – and as persistent – as the hills, as exemplified by the international colloquial term for insanity or madness: lunacy in English; lunatique in French; mondsucht in German; lunatico in Italian. The Holy Bible, the Talmud and the Koran all refer to the association between the moon and epilepsy, a belief that was shared by Aristotle, Ptolemy and Galen, the medical dictator of the Roman Empire whose teachings dominated western practice for nigh on a millenium and a half.

Today, popular belief in the effect of the moon is still widespread. As one German writer has put it: 'The Bedouin says that it is not well to gaze fixedly at the moon; French peasants consider it dangerous to sleep in the moonlight; mothers in this country are still careful to pull down the shades and shut out the moonlight from the children's bedrooms. Among Brazilian

Indians, mothers, immediately after delivery, hide themselves and their babies in the thickest part of the forest to prevent moonlight from reaching them.'

The poets, so often the mirror of popular beliefs, have commemorated the belief, as Shakespeare does in *Othello*:

> It is the very error of the moon;
> She comes more nearer earth than she has wont,
> And makes men mad.

Milton not only propagated the association, in *Paradise Lost*:

> Demoniac frenzy, moping melancholy,
> And moon-struck madness,

he also believed, like Chatterton, that his intellect was more vigorous during the phase of the full moon, while in the world of painting Raphael dramatically delineated the association in the 'Moonstruck Boy'.

Even today the belief dies hard. In his intriguing essay on 'Mania and The Moon', published in the *Psychoanalytical Review* in 1958, Dr Douglas Kelley records a psychiatric visitor to the Windward Islands in 1936 as saying: 'The guard who took me around told me that the insane, male and female, were generally easy to handle, except about the time of the full moon when special precautions had to be taken in order to restrain them.' On which Dr Kelley's comment is: 'This belief is prevalent in the United States, and many mental hospital nurses and attendants will vouch for the fact that they can tell the period of the full moon by the increasing excitement and loss of sleep of patients who become more disturbed at this time.' Even more interesting is his note that in the United States in 1938 'a defendant was permitted to plead guilty to a reduced charge on the plea of his attorney that "he suffers periodic 'mental explosions' especially when the moon is full".'

Dr Kelley is not impressed by the mass of evidence he produces and reaches the conclusion that 'on the basis of evidence determined to date there is no support for the belief that the light of the full moon affects the psychiatric or healthy in a way different from light of any other source.' What he does not exclude, or even mention, is the possibility that other meteorological changes occurring at different phases of the moon may have an effect on the mind – or body.

Before leaving these lunar regions, and as a lead-in to the subject of suicide and the weather, it may be noted that reports from Texas, covering a three-year period and 2497 suicides and 2017 homicides, revealed 'no significant relationship between the phases of the moon, or sunspots on the one hand, and the incidence of suicide or homicide on the other. Neither was there any relationship with geomagnetic fluctuations.' A more detailed study of the suicides and homicides in Houston, Texas, during one year, in which their relationship to eleven weather variables (temperature, wind speed, wind direction, barometric pressure, relative humidity, visibility, ceiling height, rain, fog, thunderstorms, and cloudiness), was equally fruitless in tracking down any association.

This, however, is clearly not the whole story, as turning back the pages of time for seven decades will show. In 1908, the *Journal of the American Medical Association* published a leading article noting that 'three of the best authorities' on suicide – drawn from Prussia, Paris and St Petersburg – had reached the conclusion that in Europe suicides invariably attained their maximum incidence in June and their lowest incidence in December. It also noted a report that in New York the suicide rate is 'most marked on the clearest, sunniest and pleasantest days [of spring and summer]. The clear dry days show the greatest number of suicides and the wet, partly cloudy days the least, and with differences too great to be attributed to accident or chance.'

This caught the eye of *The Lancet*, which in an annotation proceeded to explain the 'apparent contradiction' of suicide being most common in fine weather, as opposed to the traditional view, on the principle of the contrast between mood and weather. This is now quoted more or less *in extenso* as a delightful example of old-fashioned dialectics, so sadly lacking in these days of ephemeral argument. On 'dull days', *The Lancet* propounded, 'at least the elements are in keeping with his feelings. A black firmament is as fitting a background for the disconsolate mind as is the shrieking blast for Lear's despair . . . On bright days the despairing man not only sees all rejoicing but he may well think that every fellow-creature whom he meets is rejoicing in harmony; he and he alone is utterly wretched and miserable. When everything looked grey around him and everybody was grumbling things were not quite intolerable, but there is no place for him in a laughing world and he had best be out of it at once.'

This in turn produced a letter from a layman, in which, based on his own experience stretching over a decade, he demonstrated that both journals were wrong, and that suicide is associated with barometric depression and not sunshine.

'In the case of a particularly sensitive and highly strung temperament such as is mine unfortunately,' he wrote, 'there is some part of the brain that is extremely sensitive to variations in barometric changes or some other influence not yet discovered.' 'I believe', he continued, 'in my case and in thousands of others in varying degrees certain brain centres act simply as a far more sensitive and delicate barometric instrument than the ordinary barometer. I invariably foretell a coming change for the better or worse not a few hours ahead but three days to as much as ten days ahead. I have never yet been known to be wrong in this matter and I can not only state with precision the time of the coming change but also the duration of the change and its relative intensity . . . The manner in which I am able to foretell the weather changes is simply this. I have learned that I invariably feel what is known as mental depression, slight or severe, and the reverse as the case may be, in advance of weather changes. The depression comes on rapidly, sometimes suddenly, and sometimes very gradually. It may last for only a few minutes, for hours, and sometimes for a day or a little more . . . I have no reason to believe that I am alone in this special weather sensitiveness . . . The periods of suicidal tendency will coincide with about three or four days in advance of atmospheric depressions coming on during finer weather conditions of the atmosphere.'

A more logical, precise statement it would be difficult to evolve. How true it is of suicides as a whole it is impossible to say but, in view of the other stresses and strains involved in evoking the act of self-destruction, it is unlikely that we shall ever fathom the precise role of climate in this still all too common tragedy of life.

Inevitably the possible correlation of the psychoses, including schizophrenia, with climate changes has attracted attention. As far as back as 1935, a German report, based on 40 000 cases observed over four years, 'demonstrated graphically', in the words of a New York psychiatrist, 'a clearly observable relationship between the sixty-seven magnetic storms during this time and the incidence of nervous and mental diseases and suicides', ominously adding, however, that these results 'were not subjected to statistical treatment.' In an article in *Nature* in 1963, this psychiatrist and his colleagues, on the basis of a correlation of 28 642 admissions to New York mental hospitals and 'magnetic storms' between July 1957 and October 1961, reported that 'a significant relationship has been shown between psychiatric disturbance as reflected in hospital admissions and natural magnetic storms'. Two years later, in a subsequent report based on a study of schizophrenic patients, they somewhat modified their views. The correlation was now with cosmic ray ranges, not the whole range of geomagnetic activity. It was claimed, however, that 'statistically significant relationships of striking magnitude between cosmic ray indexes and mood behaviour can be observed in the majority of schizophrenic patients, particularly when the ratings are made one to two days after the geophysical event.'

An interesting follow-up to these reports was carried out two years later by a Canadian psychologist who, over a three-month period (January to April) correlated what he described as the 'self-evaluated mood reports' (four a day) of ten students with ten meteorological-geophysical variables, including geomagnetic activity. What is described as 'an interesting trend' was noted of 'a small but consistent negative correlation between mood reports and geomagnetic activity.' The over-all impression – and it would not be justifiable to use any stronger word such as 'conclusion' – was that 'higher' moods tended to occur more often in the first and second days after 'sunny days', whilst 'lower' moods were preceded by cloudy days typified by high but consistent relative humidity. Which is more or less what one would expect. Most of us feel better and brighter on a sunny day and somewhat 'low' on dull days – perhaps even more so during those long dark early days of the new year.

We are here verging on the difficult territory of the personal factor in deciding to what extent our complaints are due to the weather and the extent to which they may be an indirect effect through the mind. Lord Nuffield provides a classical example of this confused picture. In a letter in *The Times* in June 1977, the Emeritus Professor of Clinical Medicine in Oxford University, referred to 'the charming old house inside the works near the corner of the road at Temple Cowley where Lord Nuffield had his office for the whole of the latter part of his life'. This house, it was suggested, should be preserved and 'with it should be preserved the wind vane connected with a pointer and dial in his office, on which Lord Nuffield kept a watchful eye, for like Mr Jarmdyce he believed that he was subject to an uncomfortable sensation when the wind was in the east.'

This interested me and I wrote to Professor L. J. Witts and asked him if he could elucidate the problem. In the course of his reply he wrote: 'He [Lord Nuffield] used to get some sacro-iliac [low-back] pain and it would not be unnatural to believe it was worse when the wind was in the east. Apart from this – indeed I don't think he had any special treatment apart from a sun lamp – I think he merely thought that the wind is in the east, that's why I'm feeling low.' 'After all,' Professor Witts concluded his letter, with the shrewd comment that will be echoed by every wise doctor, 'most of us feel better if we can be given some plausible explanation for our symptoms.' A factor that must be borne in mind in considering climate and the mind.

We are on much firmer ground when we come to consider the effect of heat on the mind. For long the condition known as tropical neurasthenia, or tropical fatigue, has been recognised as one of the hazards of life in the tropics for white people. Undoubtedly there was often an underlying neurotic basis but even the most stolid of personalities could crack up mentally, or at least emotionally, under the climatic stresses of hot tropical climes. For this various factors are to blame. As Professor Burch has pointed out: 'There are psychological as well as physical differences between man living in a tropical climate and man living in a temperate climate. In the tropics where the climate varies little from day to day, the monotony of the weather produces a mental lassitude in which initiative and creative thought are impaired. By contrast, in a temperate climate with rapidly changing barometric pressures and stormy days followed by clear sunny days, man is energetic, imaginative and creative.' In other words, climatically, variety is the spice of life. In addition, however, to quote Professor Burch again, 'hot and humid atmospheres produce psychic stress.' 'Part of this stress', he notes, 'is related simply to sensations of discomfort. In some instances the cerebral brain circulation may be reduced. The ability to think clearly and to concentrate is impaired. Psychasthenia and neurasthenia develop rapidly. Errors in solving problems are made by persons working under stressful conditions.'

This is why it is so important to submit all candidates for service in the tropics to careful psychological assessment as was done in the case of officer candidates during the 1939–45 War. Any evidence of emotional immaturity or instability, or mental instability, almost automatically acts as a bar to tropical service. Once accepted, it is important that periods of service should be frequently broken by periods of furlough, and all new arrivals, especially if sent up country, should be carefully watched for signs of incipient breakdown. Not the least useful standard of assessment here is the consumption of alcohol. One reason why the old missionaries were able to carry on for much longer periods in the tropics without home leave was their religious faith and their teetotalism.

Teetotalism may not be essential for healthful living in the tropics, but the 'sundowner', excellent tranquilliser though it may be in moderation, can be a real snare and delusion for the harassed unstable personality, and many a successful career has foundered on this medical hazard of tropical climes. Fortunately, recovery is often the rule on transfer home, but once an individual has shown sufficient signs of tropical psychic stress to require return to the home country, he should never be posted again to the tropics.

Typical of the various experiments carried out to demonstrate the effect of high temperature is that in which the performance of twelve volunteers in an adding test and in a test requiring prolonged vigilance was measured at normal body temperature and when their temperature was raised to $101 \cdot 3°$ F. ($38 \cdot 5°$ C.). Compared with the performance at normal temperature, at the higher temperature the ability to add was impaired, but vigilance was improved. Equally interesting was the fact that though in other ways the volunteers became acclimatised to their repeated exposure to the hot humid conditions used to raise their temperatures, there was no improvement in their ability to add. In other words, there was no 'short-term adaptation of the central nervous system functions tested to repeated elevations of temperature.' Like all these somewhat artificial tests carried out in the laboratory, such results must be accepted with caution, as they differ in many respects from conditions actually pertaining 'in the field'. Thus, it is possible that the improvement in vigilance was the result of the volunteers realising that they were under trial and therefore striving to do their best. On the other hand, it is of interest that, in spite of this increased vigilance, their ability to add was consistently impaired.

There is evidence, however, that these effects of climate on the mind may in certain cases be the result of an increase of positive air ions, which is induced by certain weather fronts. This is a subject that has been intensively studied by Dr Sulman and his colleagues in Hebrew University, Jerusalem. In Israel the common cause of what is variously known as tropical lethargy, or the exhaustion syndrome, is the hot dry wind, Sharav, which afflicts the country annually. According to Dr Sulman and his colleagues, around a third of the population of Israel are affected by this wind, complaining of apathy, depression, fatigue, lack of concentration, confusion and sleeplessness. Sharav, it is claimed – and the evidence is impressive – is preceded by a weather front, the electrical changes of which include an excess of positive air ions. It is these, they contend, that cause the mental and emotional changes by inducing the release in the body of a neurohormone known as serotonin which is responsible for these changes. Among the evidence presented is the claim that around three-quarters of these patients affected by Sharav are relieved by treatment with negative air ions, that are known to antagonise the action of positive air ions. Further, psychiatric patients show an exacerbation of their symptoms on Sharav days and their needs for tranquillising increases considerably. Equally impressive is the report from Haifa that candidates for office jobs, technological jobs and technological institutes tested on Sharav days had 'higher scores for neuroticism and extroversion, and scored significantly lower than controls in intelligence tests and mechanical comprehension.'

Though there is no direct correlation between air ionisation and electrical storms characterised by thunder and lightning, it is relevant to note here that there is both clinical and experimental evidence that man and animals are affected psychologically by such electrical storms. So far as man is concerned, a certain amount of this is indirect and due to fear of the storm, but there is more to it than this. Typical of the animal experiments is that in which rats recently trained to run a maze were exposed to electromagnetic conditions resembling a lightning storm. This was found to disturb the ability of the rats to perform their recently learned task, though the effect was found to be reversible within half-an-hour. Of the observations on man, one of the most interesting is a French report of psychomotor disturbances in air-crews when their planes were struck by lightning. These consisted of 'a slowing of thought processes and psychomotor reactions', from which recovery occurred within a brief period.

Finally there falls for consideration the effect of high altitude on the mind. The behavioural changes induced by high altitude, such as deterioration of memory and judgment and the ability to perform discrete motor tasks, have been extensively described since the early days of the Spanish conquest of Peru. Other manifestations that have been reported are insomnia, lassitude, mental fatigue, irritability and euphoria, all of which could be produced by a lack of oxygen, which, of course, is the major climatic hazard of high altitudes. Even at relatively moderate heights, such as 8500 feet (2600 metres) there may be such behavioural disturbances which, though transitory, may be sufficient to impair performance, and studies of the electrical activity of the brain (electroencephalography) have shown definite changes during adaptation to high altitudes.

In this context it is of interest that in his report on the Himalayan Scientific and Mountaineering Expedition of 1960–61, which spent eight months at heights ranging from 15 000 to 19 000 feet (4570 to 5790 metres) Dr L. G. C. Pugh noted that, though 'the party appeared to acclimatise well to 19 000 feet and card-sorting and other psychological tests revealed no evidence of mental impairment, the party were mentally and physically tired.' His impression was that 19 000 feet was too high for complete adjustment and that 17 000 feet, and in some cases 15 000 feet, would be nearer the limit for plainsmen living at altitude. This fits in with the state of affairs in the Andes, where the native miners live at 17 500 (5330 metres) and climb daily to their work at 19 000 feet (5790 metres). They refused to occupy a camp built for them at 19 000 feet for longer than six weeks, on the grounds of loss of sleep and inability to enjoy food.

Dr Pugh's reference to card-sorting tests stimulated his

colleagues at the Medical Research Council to repeat the same test on eleven research scientists in Cambridge. They reported a definite increase in the number of errors at 19 000 feet, compared with sea-level. On which they comment: 'So far as we know this is the first time that a statistically reliable change in performance has been reported in men during acclimatisation at such heights.'

The latest report on this subject is that from the Indian Amy Medical Services already referred to in chapter 5, based on a study of Indian troops at altitudes ranging from 12 100 to 18 200 feet (3692 to 5538 metres). According to this report, general mental efficiency was slightly impaired on arrival at high altitudes, mental concentration and depression were somewhat increased throughout the period of stay at high altitudes, but there was no trend towards neurotic or psychotic tendencies or emotional instability. Depression was attributed to the monotony of the surroundings, and anxiety, which did not manifest itself until after eighteen months, was related to domestic affairs. The over-all conclusion was that, 'although the outgoingness or zeal for active social participation may decline during the first month of stay at high altitude, acceptance of an individual by his group members is not adversely affected. The interpersonal relationships remain congenial.' But how much of this is a tribute to the leadership?

The lower incidence of psychiatric disease recorded at high altitude, it is suggested, is linked to animal experiments which indicate that at high altitudes the brain is able to adjust itself and function satisfactorily on the available oxygen.

No account of climate and psyche would be complete without at least a reference to one of the most fascinating aspects of high altitude psychology. This is the 'hallucination' that inspired T. S. Eliot to write in *The Waste Land*:

> 'Who is the third man who walks beside you?
> When I count, there are only you and I together
> But when I look ahead up the white road
> There is always another one walking beside you.'

In *Everest 1933*, by Hugh Ruttledge, Frank Smythe records how, when climbing alone at 27 400 feet (8350 metres) after the sudden illness of Eric Shipton, his intended companion, 'all the time that I was climbing alone I had a strong feeling that I was accompanied by a second person. This feeling was so strong that it completely eliminated all loneliness I might otherwise have felt.' In the *British Medical Journal* in 1976, Dr Charles Clarke, the medical officer to the 1975 British Everest Expedition, recorded that Doug Scott and Dougal Haston, after their conquest of Everest, spent the night huddled in a snow hole, without oxygen, at 28 600 feet (8800 metres). On arrival at Camp 2 at 22 000 feet (6700 metres) they 'told of a curious sensation that a third person had been sharing the hole during the night.'

In the subsequent correspondence attention was drawn to the fact that on his solo descent from the summit of Naga Parbat (over 26 000 feet (8000 metres)) in the successful German expedition of 1953, Herrman Buhl, who was climbing without oxygen, described how he was aware of a companion advising him that he had dropped his gloves, but when he turned to speak to him there was no-one there. The physician to the expedition ascribed this 'hallucination' to the effect of lack of oxygen on the brain. Another reader, however, commented: 'I have personal experience of similar hallucinations in situations of sustained physical and mental strain at the relatively low altitudes experienced in the European Alps, and judging by comments from other mountaineers this is an accepted phenomenon of mild hypothermia, especially when associated with high altitude.'

This suggested association with hypothermia (low temperature) would explain why the same phenomenon was recorded by Sir Ernest Shackleton in his crossing of South Georgia. In his book, *South*, he wrote: 'I know that during the long march of thirty-six hours over the unnamed mountains and glaciers of South Georgia, it often seemed to me that we were four, not three. And Worsley and Crean had the same idea.'

So there we must leave unanswered T. S. Eliot's riddle: 'Who is the third man who walks beside you?'. A figment of the imagination, but how induced? By physical or psychological processes? Is it the yearning for companionship? But then, why does it occur when there are two or more in the party? Is it one's *alter ego*? As one plunges ever more deeply into the unfathomable reaches of the mind, the possibilities become ever more intriguing. Climate and psyche promise to become the 'open sesame' to untold wonders and mysteries.

19

Climate and old age

The two extremes of life – infancy and old age – are particularly
vulnerable to climatic changes, especially extremes of temperature.
Each winter in the British Isles old people die at home as the result
of cold. Accidental hypothermia occurs even in apparently fit old
folk and has been described as 'a common domestic disorder of the
elderly'. It is defined as a deep body temperature (that is, a
temperature recorded in the rectum, or by a thermistor in the ear)
below 95° F. (35° C.), and it has been estimated that around half a
million old people in Britain are at risk of hypothermia. In how
many of these it proves fatal is not known. In 1976, in England and
Wales it was given as the cause of death on only 600 death
certificates, but there is good reason to believe that even in a mild
winter as many as 55 000 deaths could be attributed to heart
attacks, strokes and infections brought on by the cold.

One of the main causes of hypothermia is that old folk cannot
maintain their body temperature because they lose heat through
their skin. Normally, on exposure to cold the blood-vessels of the
skin are reflexly constricted. This is a powerful mechanism for
conserving heat as it reduces the heat conductivity of the skin to
that of cork, once used to plug thermos flasks for this reason. This
mechanism does not come into play as effectively in the elderly as
in younger people. Thus, in one investigation in London it was

found that, though living in cooler rooms, old people with low deep body temperatures had warmer hand temperatures than old folk with normal deep body temperatures. Thus, as the authors of the report express it, 'they appeared to be exhibiting some degree of thermoregulatory failure or inadequate response to cooler surroundings.' The conditions under which this particular group of old folk (over a thousand) was living is exemplified by the fact that in over three-quarters of their houses the morning temperature was under 70°F. (21·1°C.), which is the temperature recommended by the Department of Health and Social Security, whilst in ten per cent it was below 53·6°F. (12°C.).

Even living under reasonably warm conditions, old people with heart or lung disease, especially the latter, are particularly vulnerable to cold climatic conditions. Not only does every winter bring its toll of deaths from chronic bronchitis and heart disease in the elderly, far more experience an exacerbation of their chronic bronchitis or their failing heart finds it difficult to tide them over to another spring. Even more dangerous than cold is atmospheric pollution as manifested by fog or smog, or at least the combination of the two. The onset of fog in the winter is a warning to Darby and Joan to seal all windows and stay in the warmth of their own fireside (or its modern equivalent) until the fog has dispersed.

As prevention is always better than cure, the elderly should obviously take avoiding action by ensuring that they maintain a reasonable body temperature. The first obvious measure is that they should wear adequate insulating clothing indoors as well as outdoors. As half the heat lost from a clothed adult is from the head, there is much to be said for the elderly reviving the old habit of wearing nightcaps, smoking caps (or skullcaps) and mutches. They should also follow the current fashion for wearing a fur hat out of doors. They should wear long underwear or combinations, gloves or mittens by day and bed socks by night, and have extra warm blankets on their beds. In this last respect, the metallised 'space blankets' on sale for mountaineers have much in their favour as they are light as well as efficient. An electric blanket is a *sine qua non* for the elderly. The old-fashioned hot water bottle does not give that over-all warmth that, apart from anything else, is so often the best preventative of insomnia in the elderly. A modern alternative to the conventional electric blanket is the low-wattage electric under-blanket specially designed so that it can be kept on continuously at a low heat output and is waterproof and electrically safe.

Basic to all these, of course, is an adequately heated house, not forgetting, as is so often the case, the bedroom. Central heating should be the aim, giving an equable warm clime throughout the whole house. For those who cannot afford to keep their homes adequately heated (an admittedly increasingly expensive luxury in the modern Welfare State) additional supplementary benefits are available for extra heating. Details of these can be obtained from local offices of the Department of Health and Social Security.

In these days of tranquillisers a final word of warning must be given of their potential danger in old folk in cold weather. They are liable to produce dangerous hypothermia because they directly depress the body temperature by causing vasodilatation of the blood-vessels of the skin and by abolishing shivering: two of the most certain methods that could be devised of ensuring that an old person should lose the maximum of precious body heat and thereby pass into the dangerous state of hypothermia. Further, as one of our most experienced geriatricians has pointed out, 'the degree of exposure to cold need not be severe in these patients, who can indeed become hypothermic while lying in bed.'

Excessive heat can be just as treacherous for the elderly as excessive cold. Every year heat waves bring their toll of deaths among the elderly. Typical of such episodes is that recorded in *The Times* of 28 July 1977. 'This July has been the hottest the United States has experienced since the dust bowl years of the 1930s . . . Last week New York experienced a day when the mercury rose to 104° F., only two degrees short of its highest temperature ever recorded . . . New York's death rate last week jumped by 10 per cent, hospitals reporting that many old people were overcome by an "atmospheric inversion" causing "unacceptable levels of pollution".' Again it is those with failing hearts who are most susceptible. Many an old body is just 'ticking over' so far as his heart is concerned, and any extra strain may upset this delicate balance and produce manifestations of a failing heart, such as shortness of breath, dropsy or palpitations. This is fundamentally due to slowness of adaptation to heat on the part of the elderly. Thus, in one experiment the response to increased heat was studied in ten healthy inmates of a local authority hostel (aged 65 to 80) and eight medical students (aged 20 to 24). In both there was a rise in deep body temperature but this was significantly greater in the old folk. In somewhat technical jargon this was attributed to 'delays in the initiation of behavioural responses'. One of these 'behavioural responses' is sweating, one of the body's major defences against the hazards of overheating. As described in chapter 7, unless we can sweat freely heatstroke is inevitable. In one investigation carried out in London it was found that in fourteen out of nineteen people over the age of 70 the sweating response to the injection of a drug known to induce sweating was minimal or absent. An interesting corollary was that 'it was notable that the texture and appearance of the skin of the elderly subjects with good or moderate sweating responses appeared more youthful, elastic and less wrinkled to the naked eye than of those whose sweat response was poor or absent.' For once apparently appearances were not deceptive.

The practical implications of this poor response of the ageing heart to heat is that old folk should not travel to the tropics. If possible they should live in an equable relaxing clime in a house which can be protected from excessive sunshine and have adequate means of ventilation. In hot climes some form of air conditioning is advisable but this is seldom required in the British Isles. On the other hand the house should be adequately shaded with venetian blinds and sunshades on sun-exposed windows. Clothing should be light physically and colorometrically, bedrooms should be adequately ventilated, and for the ladies there is much to be said for the delightful old parasol. Alternatively, a wide-brimmed straw hat should be worn. There is much to be said for the traditional siesta – with the feet up; nothing is a better preventative of that swelling of the ankles which is such a burden and worry to old folk in hot weather. The diet, which should be light and non-spiced, should include ample 'soft' drinks. Alcohol should be consumed in moderation, and preferably not during the heat of the day. There is much to be said for the old custom of not touching 'hard' liquor until sundown.

One final warning may be appended. Obesity, which is even more of a health hazard in hot climes than in temperate zones, is a particular hazard for old people. As it has been put: 'Men who are stoutly built are at a disadvantage in heat and more likely to have heatstroke.' The excessive fat underneath the skin interferes with the exchange of heat, encouraging retention of it and discouraging loss of it. We have all seen the wellnigh apoplectic old man becoming redder and redder, more and more uncomfortable, and more and more distressed as the temperature rose. Sooner or later something is likely to go, whether it be the heart, or one of the arteries to the brain resulting in a stroke. Slimness should therefore be the aim of the elderly. If this is not achievable, then in hot weather their movements must be as lackadaisical as possible.

20

Climate and retirement

In the case of the healthy, climate may not be as important a factor where retirement is concerned as is to the unhealthy. Nevertheless it is one that cannot be ignored. By the time retirement comes one's physical capacities are beginning to run down. To what extent this has occurred varies considerably, depending largely upon how physically active one has been in the past. The man whose exercise has merely been a mild mixture of walks, swimming in the holidays, and gardening, with no passion for, or devotion to, one particular form of sport is most easily satisfied on retirement. On the other hand, the keen golfer, climber, yachtsman, or gardener must obviously take his sport or hobby into consideration in reaching the final conclusion as to where to retire to.

Always to be remembered, of course, in the case of the married couple is that the views of the spouse must be given equal consideration. In few aspects of married life is conjugal collusion more essential than in deciding where the evening of life is to be spent. There must obviously be give and take; and the wife of the golfing enthusiast will obviously recognise that the new home must be within reasonable access of a golf course to the husband's liking, whilst the husband of a gardening enthusiast will equally recognise that the new home must possess a garden to his wife's liking and, just as important these days, within her physical capacity to manage without outside help – or at least with a minimum of that most inflated cost these days: human labour. Gone are the days of 'a labourer being worthy of his hire'. Today it is a case of the labourer insisting on the maximum he can receive for the minimum he needs to give.

Never to be forgotten is that after the age of sixty-five – the traditional age of retirement, chosen for no good reason known to the medical profession – one's physical capacities tend to slow up (or down) in a steadily increasing crescendo. Which in effect means that a site must be chosen for retirement that is not likely to be physically exhausting in the years to come. A hilly area, for instance, where it is impossible to get anywhere without climbing is to be avoided. Similarly, climatic hazards like persistent unpleasant winds are to be avoided, and for the sun-lover the amount of sunshine must be taken into consideration. The more drastic hazards, such as flooding rivers and sea–flooding must also be borne in mind. A riverside cottage seen in blazing June may seem the perfect retreat for old age, but the same cottage under a foot or more of stinking flood water is another matter.

The foot of certain valleys must also be regarded with some suspicion. 'Valleys', it has been said, 'can generate their own local winds' which, even on clear spring and summer nights, can produce a thick morning mist ensheathing the unfortunate inhabitants of the valley while the nearby hill tops are in brilliant sunshine. How often did I see this on my wartime expeditions in Surrey on the A3 between Hurtmore Corner (or Jackson's Corner as it was known locally, after one of a trilogy of brothers who played a by no means unimportant part in the development of Guildford between the two wars) and the Hog's Back – bathed in brilliant morning sunshine while down in the valley Compton with its Watts Gallery was invisibly wrapped in thick mist. A lovely picture for those looking down on it, but a somewhat depressing experience for the inhabitants of Compton.

Again, some may prefer the maximum of warmth and sunshine,

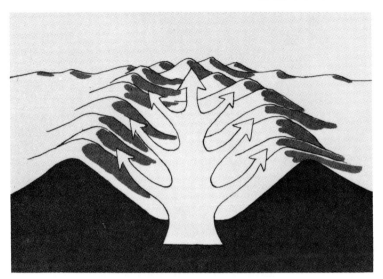

Slope winds move up a valley during the afternoon hours.

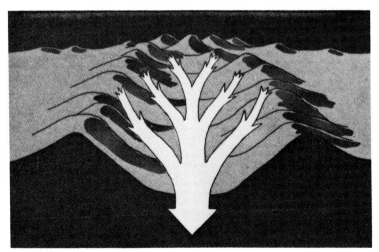

At night, sinking of cooler air reverses the wind's flow.

whilst others will prefer a reasonably exposed situation with a good healthy blow. Some prefer to be shut in or sheltered amid trees, whilst others want a view of God's wide-open spaces, without which they feel definitely claustrophobic.

These are but some of the climatic factors that must be taken into consideration in deciding the site of one's retirement. In this imperfect world where more and more seems to depend upon income (and/or capital), there may be few who can find a home for retirement that satisfies all these climatic criteria – and I am the first to admit that peace of mind, not to forget that 'peace of God which passeth all understanding', can be obtained under anything but ideal physical conditions – and of the two, peace of mind and spirit are much more important than anything else, but the ideal must always be borne in mind in reaching the final compromise. To summarise – or some might say generalise – the ideal climatic house is one built on the south-facing slope of a reasonably wide valley, not too near the bottom (like Compton), with evergreen trees to the north to provide protection and some shelter from the icy blasts of winter, and deciduous trees to the south to provide shade in the summer but no obstruction to winter sunshine when their leaves have fallen in the autumn. All on a well-drained soil. The pros and cons of heavy clay and light sandy soils are too intricate for discussion here.

For those who are victims of some chronic conditions, such as rheumatism, heart or lung disease, the choice is to a certain extent easier. The first essential is that there should be a reasonable doctor within easy access as well as an adequate hospital. The retired couple may hope that such services may not be needed too often but, when necessary, they are of vital importance. The second consideration is whether any move should be made at all. If one has a comfortable home, with all requisite medical facilities well tested over the years and within easy access, why move? Apart from anything else, friends are more important to the invalid than to the healthy citizen. To be ill without visitors can be quite devastating, and in a new town or village friends are more difficult to acquire, apart altogether from the fact that as one grows older one's capacity for developing new friendships definitely diminishes.

The sound reasons for the unfit to move are financial and medical. The old house may be too big for comfortable management, especially in these days of non-existent domestic help, or it may be too expensive to run. If therefore it is going to be a strain financially and/or physically, then a change is definitely indicated.

Medical indications depend upon the condition from which the retirer is suffering. On the whole it is a relaxing climate that is required, warm, equable, sheltered from the wind, without too much rain or cloud. Dryness of the soil as well as warmth are the two criteria for the rheumatic subject. Warmth without too cold a winter, and an absence of fog are the essentials for the chronic bronchitic subject, and very largely for the patient with an inadequate heart. Equally important in the case of the last is the absence of hills. The countryside around the house must be flat so that the optimum of exercise may be enjoyed without too much physical effort. Even in these days of the wellnigh universal internal combustion engine, easy accessibility on foot to shops, neighbours, church and social centres such as concert hall, cinema and the like is an asset. For the allergic subject freedom from the offending pollens is advisable. To a certain extent this is where the sea-coast or moderately high altitudes may be an advantage, whilst trees may be a definite handicap, especially ash, elm and oak which are among the more troublesome trees in Britain from the point of allergic reactions such as hay fever. One of the practical advantages of the sea-coast is that the predominant wind is onshore, which brings no pollen and blows away those that may be present.

One final point must be stressed. No matter how important climatic factors may be, and no matter what the illness concerned may be, the retirer, or the retiring couple, must not tear themselves up by the roots unless they are convinced that there will be sufficient compensation in the new surroundings for the loss of what has been their home in the past. To a certain extent the increasing mobility of the community has eased this problem as more and more often the roots have not had the time to sink very deeply. But even so, the final move – and for the majority of retired married couples retirement is the final move – tends to be more of a wrench.

How often in these post-war years has one seen self-made men who have made the grade to senior directorships in the Midlands decide to retire to Eastbourne or Bournemouth, convinced from their experience of summer holidays in expensive hotels there that they were the El Dorado of their dreams. Possibly they have even built their own bungalow. For a while all goes well but the boredom begins to tell. They have not sufficient aesthetic or cultural interests to occupy their minds. The wife particularly finds her new social contacts anything but forthcoming. All too often they have nothing in common. Gradually, mental deterioration creeps in and the treasure of their El Dorado becomes little more than dross.

For such people – admirable citizens as many of them are, but with no hobbies or religious faith – the wise decision would have been to stay in their old surroundings. No climatic factor, no matter how beneficial, will compensate for this pathetic – all too often tragic would be a more appropriate description – loss of interest in life, resulting in the slow death of body, mind and spirit – the antithesis of human dignity.

There remains the problem of when, if ever, there are climatic indications for retiring overseas. In general the answer is in the negative. In spite of all we say about our climate, within this island home of ours we have an almost infinite variety of climates to suit all the ills to which British man is heir. To which has to be added the definite advantage of no extremes such as tornadoes, hurricanes, earthquakes, devastating snowstorms or floods, and the like. Hitherto, we have also been free from those revolutions that have devastated so many of the climatically eligible parts of the world. Cyprus is a classical example. An ideal climate for those with chest disease, it attracted many a retired British citizen seeking, and obtaining, relief from his chronic bronchitis. But how many of these have lost their houses, and are now refugees back in the 'mother country'? Malta in a milder way shows the same effects of political disturbance on British citizens who have retired there, many of them for health reasons. Such political upheavals are bad enough for the healthy, but for the ailing they are the quintessence of bad medicine and have nothing but a deleterious effect – whatever the complaint may be, whether cardiac, respiratory or rheumatic.

Further, the upheaval of moving abroad in these days of international restrictions on the movement of money, double taxation and the like, is often too much of a strain for the ailing citizen – unless he is well enough off to be able to hand over the management of his affairs to experienced lawyers and the like.

To holiday abroad is one thing. To live abroad is quite another. In these days therefore the general medical answer to the patient asking about retiring abroad is 'No'. There are no real medical advantages compared with this country, and not a few disadvantages. If there are friends or relatives abroad that is another matter, or if there are other strong ties, cultural or otherwise, then a slightly different complexion can be put on the matter. St Leonards may not sound as exciting as St Tropez, the Isle of Wight as Cyprus, or the Channel Islands as the Canaries, but for the retired invalid they have much to be said in their favour and there is a host of witnesses to the benefit that the retired can obtain from British climes that heal.

21

Travel, climate and health

'And what should they know of England who only England know?' sang Kipling. For long, indeed up until the last few decades, the vast majority of the inhabitants of this island home of ours knew little of the lands beyond the seas from personal experience. Not only, in the words of Sir Edward Coke, was 'a man's house his castle', it was also his home where he dug in his roots, if they were not already dug in, and considered it the right and proper and enjoyable thing to spend his life there. War and commerce might take a man to the distant parts of the world, but all the time his dreams were of returning to the home of his fathers. In the nineteenth century it became fashionable for the upper and middle classes to 'do' the Continent in the great name of culture. As travel became easier, particularly following the ramification of railways, they also sought new climes to restore their ailing health. But for the majority of the populace holidays within the home country were the rule.

Today overseas travel is *de rigeur* for all sections of society, played up with their usual devilish skill by the so-called media and the advertising industry at the behest of, and to the greater financial glory of, the travel industry. Fish and chips à l'Espagnole is a much more attractive item on the menu than the same dish in the local fish and chip shop. Inevitably in these days of mass travel a not inconsiderable number of people who are medically unfit to do so are flitting about the world, causing alarm to fellow-passengers and anxiety to stewards and stewardesses. The vast majority are travelling either by air or by car. The sea is no longer looked upon as a means of holiday travel; nor are trains, except at home.

It is not the purpose of this chapter to provide a medical *vade mecum* of travel. What is proposed is to deal with some of the more important aspects in so far as they affect the health of the traveller from the climatic point of view. Inevitably most of it will deal with air travel which now claims around 500 million travellers a year.

On the relative merits of air and sea travel all that need be said so far as the invalid is concerned is that the only advantage of air travel is its speed. Even at its best it can be tiring, especially if there are stops in transit. At its worst it can be, literally and metaphorically, one of the most frustrating methods of travel. Gone are the days of individual attention on arrival at the airport of departure. Today these are all too liable to be more like bedlam than anything else, with long waits on account of weather conditions, technical hitches, or employees suddenly deciding they have a grievance that demands attention. Even if all goes well chronologically there are long queues to register and then get aboard the plane or bus. Customs formalities are dealt with in the erect position amid a seething mass of humanity all desperate to be first away, whereas on board ship or train such examinations are carried out in one's cabin or compartment. This is not intended as a caricature of Heathrow, Gatwick or any other international airport, but it does reflect the experience of many a traveller, particularly if he or she is embarking on a holiday in search of climes that heal.

For the invalid travelling by air I would recommend British Airways every time – not from any narrow chauvinistic attitude but simply because experience has shown that its medical department lays itself out to provide every facility to make the journey as comfortable as possible. It carries out careful medical clearance of elderly, sick or infirm passengers before accepting them, and for this purpose requires the completion of a medical questionnaire by the passenger's family doctor. These are personally cleared by a medical officer. In 1976, the medical officer responsible for passenger services dealt with 26 000 such cases. These regulations have recently (1978) been modified. Prospective travellers with a stable disability such as arthritis have now only to tell the airline of their condition at the time of booking. Those who have recently had a serious illness or operation still need a certificate from their doctor stating that they are fit to travel.

Should a passenger take ill in flight, every British Airways aircraft is fitted with oxygen and certain essential drugs, which is more than can be said for the planes of certain other companies. Further, should there not be a doctor on board – and it is amazing how many doctors seem to spend their time flying about the world – if the captain wishes further advice he can obtain this by means of the very long range single side-band radio now fitted to most long-range aircraft, which enables him to seek medical advice from air-line medical departments often thousands of miles away from base.

As the principal medical officer of the admirably organised British Airways Medical Service has justifiably claimed, his Department is only too pleased to help doctors with their elderly or infirm patients and to give advice if necessary. As he points out, however, 'prior warning is essential so that cabin crew and staff on the ground en route can be adequately briefed on the individual requirements.' So far as the prospective passenger is concerned, this means that he (or she) must consult his (or her) family doctor in good time – first to obtain his advice as to fitness for air travel to whatever destination is in mind, and secondly to give the family doctor plenty of time to get in touch with the air-line medical department.

The simulated altitude on modern pressurised aircraft is equivalent to 5000 to 7000 feet (1520 to 2100 metres), this being the lowest pressure that can safely be obtained. For the ordinary healthy individual this is a perfectly safe and comfortable pressure, but it may make breathing just a little difficult for the passenger with heart or lung trouble. Seldom, however, is it necessary to make use of the oxygen available on board, but it is important to realise that the breathing difficulty is of no great significance – and not panic and start over-breathing. This is only asking for trouble. If your family doctor and the air-line medical officer have accepted you as fit to travel, then there is nothing to worry about.

On the other hand, particularly on account of the pressure in the cabin, there are certain elementary rules that all passengers should observe. These are to eat sparingly throughout the trip, drink plenty of bland fluid but avoid any gaseous drinks and cut down alcohol and smoking to a minimum. The advice to drink plenty of bland, non-gaseous fluid is necessary as the modern aircraft cabin has a relatively dry atmosphere. This is particularly marked in U.S. aircraft which do not as a rule use humidifiers, which are fitted in British aircraft. In addition it is comforting to wear loose fitting clothes. This applies particularly to the ladies, in whom tight corsets and the like can produce quite considerable discomfort in flight. Two further practical pieces of advice from an experienced member of the medical staff of British Airways may be given. 'For a long journey the traveller should be advised to have two good nights' sleep before setting out.' 'Plan the flight well in advance. If possible a day flight and/or arrival in time to go to bed at a time equivalent to the bedtime at the point of departure.'

A further point to be borne in mind is that certain airports are at altitudes in excess of 5000 feet. This means that passengers with heart complaints must take things particularly slowly for a few days until they become acclimatised to the reduced availability of oxygen in the rarefied atmosphere. While on this question of patients with heart trouble, it is important to stress that they should not hesitate to ask for oxygen if they are at all breathless and this does not settle quickly. On the whole, however, as one observer has put it, 'cardiac patients tolerate air travel well unless they are severely short of breath, and may find the strain of flying less than that of a long journey involving tiring changes from ship to trains and cars.' He does, however, add a note of caution for 'travellers with a history of heart or lung disease who plan flights in underdeveloped areas of the world. It cannot be assumed that safeguards will be available. Thus in Peru some tourist flights may have to be taken in an unpressurised aircraft.' My response to which is that such patients should avoid running such risks unless the trip is absolutely essential.

While on this subject of high altitudes, a word of warning is necessary to the fit as well as the unfit. In the words of Professor D. Heath and Dr D. R. Williams in their fascinating book, *Man at High Altitude*, acute mountain sickness (see chapter 5) is 'likely to prove an increasing problem in the travel industry for the tendency for holidays to be taken in more exotic places raises the possibility of tourists being suddenly exposed to the hypoxia [low oxygen] of high altitude after rapid transit by plane from sea level . . . The traveller should not attempt to ascend from sea level to high altitudes rapidly . . . It is much better to break the journey and spend a few days at an intermediate altitude.'

That this is no idle warning was vividly demonstrated by an article in *The Times* in 1978. Entitled 'The Dizzy Heights of Everest', it was a perfect example of how not to travel. The authoress, a journalist sampling a packaged tour organised by a well-known air-line, on her own admission no climber, reached a height of 12 700 feet (3870 metres) on the third day out and collapsed with mountain sickness, for which she required oxygen. And she was not the only one, judging from her comment that the 'hotel seems like a hospital and oxygen cylinders are rushed to fellow sufferers.' Three of her seven 'tips' are worthy of note, the first because of the unsoundness of its reference to age; the second for the light it throws on the harum-scarum aura surrounding the whole episode; and the third to damn it. 'Check your health first with your doctor. Age is no deterrent, but physical condition can be.' 'Take extra cash. Oxygen costs money and a helicopter to fly you out, if you are really sick, costs £1000.' 'Take a bottle of whisky, or some other spirit. It's very warming and is difficult to buy.'

This episode is reported in some detail as a perfect example of how not to do it, and a warning against the advertising campaign for such exotic packaged holidays (price £580 to £690), of which this is presumably a prelude. It is of interest in passing to note that *The Times* resurrected some of its one-time wisdom and accompanied the article by a note from its Medical Correspondent on mountain sickness. It is his advice that should be followed by those who indulge in what the older generation of climbers would describe as the bastardisation of mountaineering: 'There is no way of predicting who will or will not be affected [by mountain sickness] and the only safe rule is to stay below 12 000 feet for the first two weeks at altitude.'

One of the problems of flying is the swelling of the feet and ankles that is liable to occur. This is by no means unique to flying. It was well recognised in the days when travel by sea was the rule, and was variously known as 'dead ankles' and 'Colombo plop'. It is largely the result of sitting for long periods with the legs in the dependent position. 'Springbok oedema', as I christened it in *The Lancet* when I first encountered it on a night flight from Johannesburg, is particularly liable to occur in people with varicose veins. To discourage its development passengers on long flights should periodically 'stretch their legs' by strolling up and down the alleyway, and, when sitting, should regularly bend and unbend their ankles. This muscular movement goes far to prevent the swelling in many. As does making a point of spending the available time at transit stops walking and not sitting. The wearing of comfortable shoes is also helpful, but I would be reluctant to follow the advice of one writer on the subject, 'to have loose fitting slippers in the night bag.' Comfortable, yes; but when you come to put on your shoes again you may find your feet so swollen that they are difficult to get on – as one good lady on my Johannesburg flight found to her cost. By all means loosen the shoes, if they are laced, but don't take them off.

Another point not widely appreciated is that it is unwise to fly within twelve hours of any dive with an aqualung, and twenty-four hours should elapse before a flight when a deep dive, i.e. over 100 feet (30 metres) has been made.

It is not proposed to give a long list of medical conditions in relation to flying, but certain guidelines may be indicated. Patients who have had an uncomplicated coronary attack are usually fit to fly in six weeks. They should be ambulant, able to walk at a reasonable pace for eighty to a hundred yards and climb ten to twelve stairs. But, no matter how fit they feel, they should not fly without first taking their family doctor's advice. Those who have had an abdominal operation should not attempt to fly for ten to fourteen days. Colostomy patients may find that their colostomy becomes over-active and should therefore be prepared with reserve dressings. Epileptics should not attempt to fly without an understanding companion, certainly not without medical permission, and the airline medical department must be notified. Pregnant ladies on long international journeys should travel by the end of the thirty-fifth week of pregnancy.

Two types of cases are unsuitable for air travel. No case of infectious disease can be accepted for travel on a scheduled aircraft, and, in the words of the Deputy Director of British Airways Medical Services, 'any mental case that may be a hazard to the safety of the aircraft and its occupants, or so repulsive in appearance as to cause distress, is not normally acceptable without special provision being made.'

The increasing extent to which passenger ships are switching to cruising is ample evidence of the extent to which the air has purloined those who formerly travelled by sea. Whether this is to the benefit of the passengers is an open question – apart from the speed factor. If there is no great hurry getting from A to B there is much to be said from the health point of view for travelling by sea. It is restful, and the process of acclimatisation to changing climes is gradual. Much depends, of course, on the weather. The five-day transatlantic run may be sheer purgatory to all except seasoned sailors. On the other hand, the voyage to South Africa, the Indian subcontinent, South-East Asia, the Far East, Australia, or South America can be, and usually is for most of the way, a comfortable trip from the point of weather. Granted that the Bay of Biscay and the Cape swell can be distinctly upsetting, but on a long voyage these are relatively short interludes.

In addition, the major shipping companies have adequate medical departments, and their ships are staffed by efficient doctors and nurses, as well as sick-bays. As in the case of flying, any invalid, incapacitated or elderly person should first consult his or her family doctor, and the appropriate medical department should be given full details so that special arrangements can be made, if necessary, to help them on board.

The same general rules apply to sea cruises. Provided the ship is owned by a reputable shipping company, two or three weeks, or longer, may be an excellent 'tonic', rest or means of convalescence. The only trouble about some of the cheaper and more popular cruises is that the 'clientele' tends to be somewhat mixed with a predominance of what is euphemistically known as 'good fellowship', but all too often means boisterous, raucous and over-drinking sessions at all hours of the day. Careful pre-selection is therefore necessary, preferably based on the personal experience of those whose tastes one shares. As in the case of sea voyages, care must be taken in the choice of cabin – that it is well ventilated and not adjacent to noisome water or steam pipes, and the like.

One final word of warning is indicated here, admirably summarised by one of the most experienced doctors in the field of travel. 'Some of the smaller mushroom shipping companies of lesser repute who may be sailing under flags of convenience frequently provide only minimal medical facilities. For the elderly or invalid, to travel with these companies is to ask for trouble. Similarly on such liners the food is frequently of poorer quality and with the type of cooking may cause intestinal upsets which are most unpleasant when a small cabin is the only place in which to be ill. Further, with this type of cruise, remaining on board when you are meant to be going on shore trips and excursions is not encouraged, which may be fatiguing for the elderly especially if the weather is hot.' This is certainly one sphere in which parsimony (and bargains) are false economy. If you cannot afford to travel in comfort – not necessarily luxury, stay at home, especially if you are proposing to travel to hot and humid climes or to relatively high altitudes. Overseas climes that heal should only be sought under conditions conducive to health and comfort.

Selected Bibliography

Chandler, T. J., and Gregory, S. *The Climate of the British Isles*, 1976, Longman.

Claiborne, Robert. *Climate, Man and History*, 1973, Angus & Robertson.

Dubos, René. *Mirage of Health*.

Heath, D., and Williams, D. R. *Man at High Altitude*, 1977, Churchill Livingstone.

Howarth, Patrick. *When The Riviera was Ours*, 1977.

Howe, G. Melvyn. *Man, Environment and Disease in Britain*, 1976, Pelican.

Inward, Richard. *Weather Lore*, 1950. E.P. Publishing Ltd.

Lawrence, J. S. *Rheumatism and Populations*, 1977, Heinemann Medical Books Ltd.

Renbourn, E. T. *Materials and Clothing in Health and Disease*, 1972.

Index

Index

Bees, 20, 26
Belly binder, 120–2
Bennet, Dr J. H., 12
Bernard, Claude, 29
Birds, influence of climate on, 19
Blood clotting, 138, 165
Blood pressure, 58, 79
Bognor Regis, 14
Boot, Jesse, 13
Bora wind, 38
Boudin, J. C. M., 6–7
Bournemouth, 14, 139, 145, 148, 206
  Pine Walk, Lower Pleasure Gardens,
   51
Bracing climes, 32–43, 49, 155
Brewster, Sir David, 34
Brigerbad, Switzerland, 57
Brighton, 14, 45
British Airways, 209–11, 214
British Everest Expedition (1975), 194
British Migraine Association, 169, 173
Bronchitis, chronic, 42, 60, 70, 96, 98,
  145–9, 154, 155, 162, 197, 205, 207
Broncho-pneumonia, 153–4, 155
Brougham, Lord, 11–12
Bruce, General C. G., 54, 55
Brynje, Captain, 124
Budleigh Salterton, 39
Buhl, Herrman, 194
Burch, Prof. G. E., 133, 134, 135, 162,
  182, 189
Burnet, Sir Macfarlane, 150
Burns, Robert, 39
Burton, Richard, 181

Cairngorms, 172
Canary Islands, 13, 14, 43, 139, 148,
  207
Cancer, 18, 93, 174–80
Cannes, 11, 34
Cape south-easter, 38–9
Carbon dioxide in atmosphere, 97, 98
Carlyle, Thomas, 108
Carnarvon, Earl of, 72, 74
Caroline, Princess of Monaco, 38
Caroline, Queen, 14

Castellamare, 4, 13
Cellular clothing, 124, 125, 126
Celsus, Aulus, 4
Chamberlain, Joseph, 92
Chandler, Prof. T. J., 95–6
Channel Islands, 13, 145, 148, 207
Chatterton, Thomas, 184
Chilblains, 66, 90–1
Children, 15, 67, 156, 177
  asthma, 140–2, 143, 144–5
  broncho-pneumonia, 153–4, 155
  clothing, 110–11
  marine climatotherapy, 48–9, 50, 51
  mountain therapy, 58–60, 61
China, 4–5, 182–3
Chlorofluorocarbons, 99
Cholera, 150
Cholera belt, 113, 120–2
Cholesterol, 138
Claiborne, Robert, xi–xii
Clarke, Dr Charles, 194
Climatron, 163
Cochrane, Peter, 74–5, 116–17
Clothes, 108–26
  children's, 110–11
  cholera belt, 120–2
  insulation of, 123–4
  materials used for, 122–3
  neckwear, 124–5, 126
  night, 105–5
  old people's, 197, 199–200
  spinal pad, 118–19
  swaddling, 109, 110
  topi, 113, 114, 115–18
Coke, Sir Edward, 208
Cold weather: adaptation to, 18–19,
  28–9
  asthma and, 141, 142–4
  chronic bronchitis and, 146–7
  clothing for, 111, 120, 125
  hazards of, 64–70
  heart disease and, 128, 129, 130–1,
   132–3
  infection and, 152–3, 155, 156
  rheumatism and, 163–5, 167
Colds *see* Infection

220

Index

Heart disease, 14, 42, 48, 58, 60, 70, 78, 96, 127–39, 162, 197, 198–9, 200, 204, 210, 211–12

Heat: adaptation to, 19, 28
clothing and, 112, 113–19, 121, 124–5
effect on the mind, 189–91
effect on old people, 198–200
hazards of hot climes, 71–82
heart disease and, 128, 129–30, 132, 133–7
see also Sunshine

Heat cramps, 77

Heatstroke, 71–2, 74–5, 77, 79–81, 83–5, 115, 200

Heat waves, heart failure caused by, 133–4, 135, 136–7, 198–9

Heath, Prof D., 212

Heberden, William, 150

High altitudes, 17, 21, 158
air travel, 209–14
asthma and, 143–4, 145
effect on man, 52–8
effect on the mind, 192–5
mountain therapy, 58–63
retirement at, 205
rheumatism and, 165
see also Everest

Hill, Sir Leonard, iv, 32–3, 48, 55, 64–5, 72, 108, 111, 112, 113–15, 116, 122–3, 143, 167

Himalayan Scientific and Mountaineering Expedition, 192

Hippocrates, 127–8, 130

Hippocratic School of medicine, 2–3, 4

Hirsch, Augustus, 6

Holidays: for asthmatic people, 141, 145
mountain, 60–2, 212–13
sea cruises, 215
seaside, 51

Homicide, 185

Hormones, 30, 55, 66
role in determining skin colour, 86–7

Hot water bottle, 198

House of Commons, ventilation of, 113

Hoverflies, 20

Howarth, Patrick, 12

Huang (Hwang Ti), Emperor of China, 4–5

Humidifiers, 211

Humidity, 21, 68
asthma and, 141, 142, 144
chronic bronchitis and, 145, 146
damp cold, 69–70
heart disease and, 128, 133–4, 135–7
infection and, 151, 154, 156
rheumatism and, 161, 162–3, 167–8

Huntingdon, Countess of, 45

Huntington, Ellsworthy, xi

Hyperpyrexia, 75

Hypothalamus, 175–6

Hypothermia, 65, 70, 194, 196–7, 198

Immunoglobulins, 55, 158, 165

India, 5, 193
atmospheric pollution, 96–7
high altitude research, 52–3, 58
pneumonic plague, 152–3
sola topis, 115, 116

Infection, 58, 150–9, 214

Insects, 20, 26

Insomnia, 25, 43

Inwards, Richard, 31

Ionizing radiation, 56–7

Irwin, Lord, 116

Ischaemic heart disease, 138

Isle of Wight, 39, 48, 145, 207

Jamaica, 166

Jerusalem, 144, 170, 191

Johnson, Samuel, 150

Judd, Denis, 92

Julius Caesar, 113

Kelgren, Prof. J. H., 166–7

Kelley, Dr Douglas, 184–5

Keswick, 14

Kingsley, Charles, 1, 3

Kipling, Rudyard, 208

Lawrence, Dr J. S., 166, 167

Index